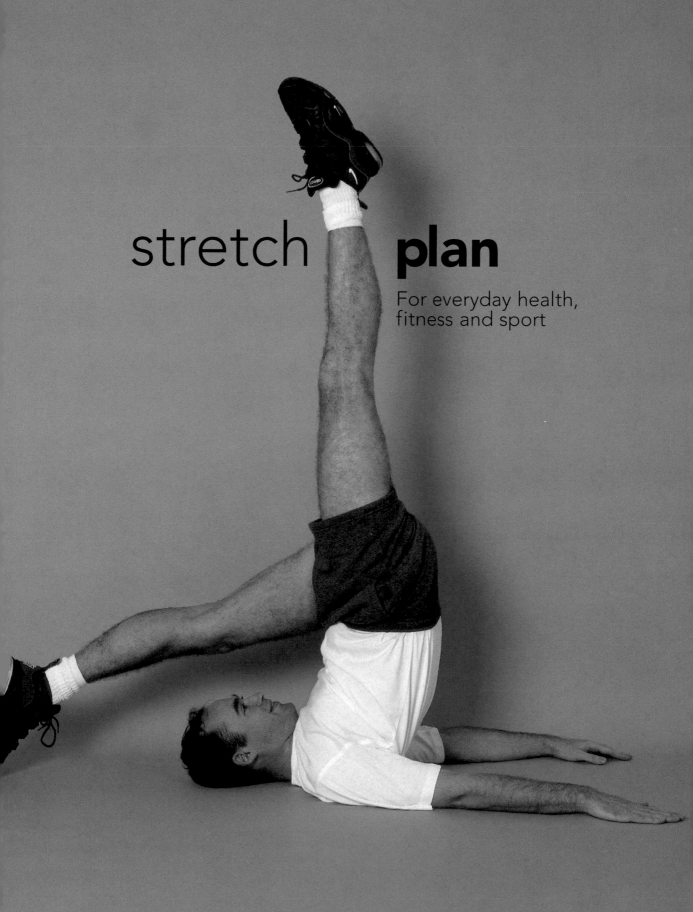

stretch **plan**

For everyday health,
fitness and sport

A CIP catalogue record for this book is available
from the British Library.

ISBN 1 84222 815 3

Executive Editor: Judith More
Art Director Penny Stock
Photography: Susanna Price and Ruth Jenkinson
Design: Nick Harris
Copy Editor: Jonathan Hilton
Production: Janette Burgin

Printed and bound in Dubai

The publishers would like to thank the following companies for
their generosity in lending sports equipment for this book:
Olympus Sport, Reebok, Snow & Rock, Denver Athletic, and
Surrey Cricket Centre.

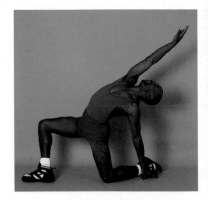

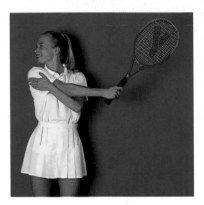

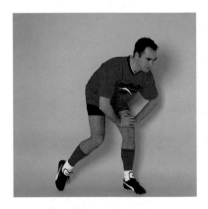

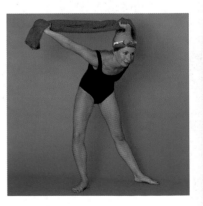

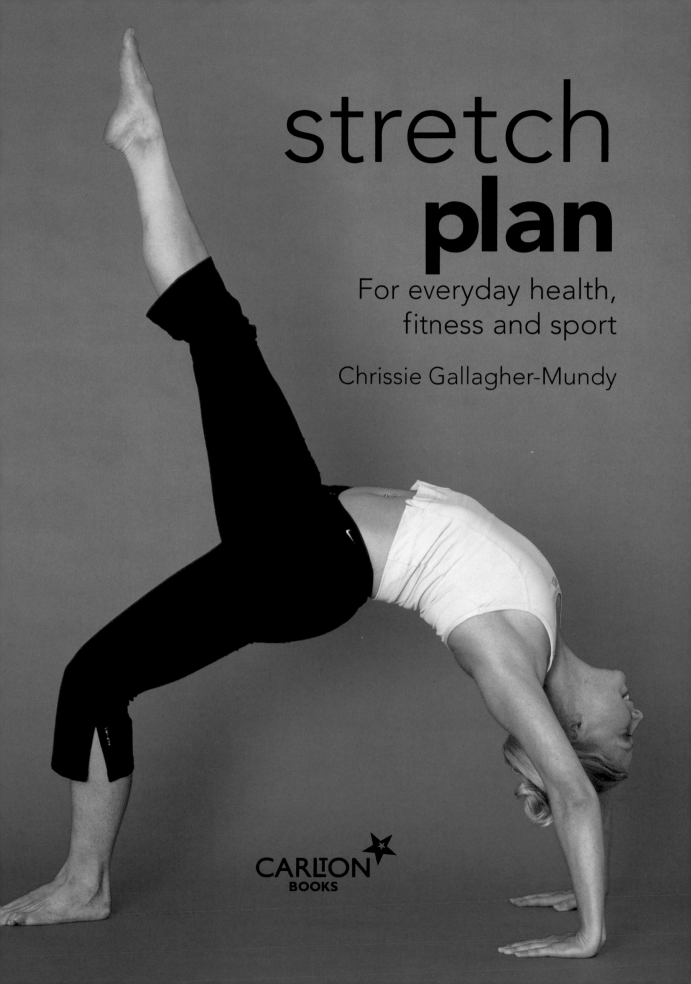

stretch
plan

For everyday health,
fitness and sport

Chrissie Gallagher-Mundy

CARLTON
BOOKS

contents

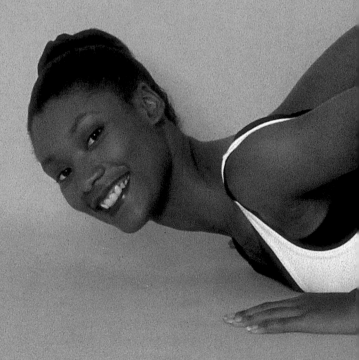

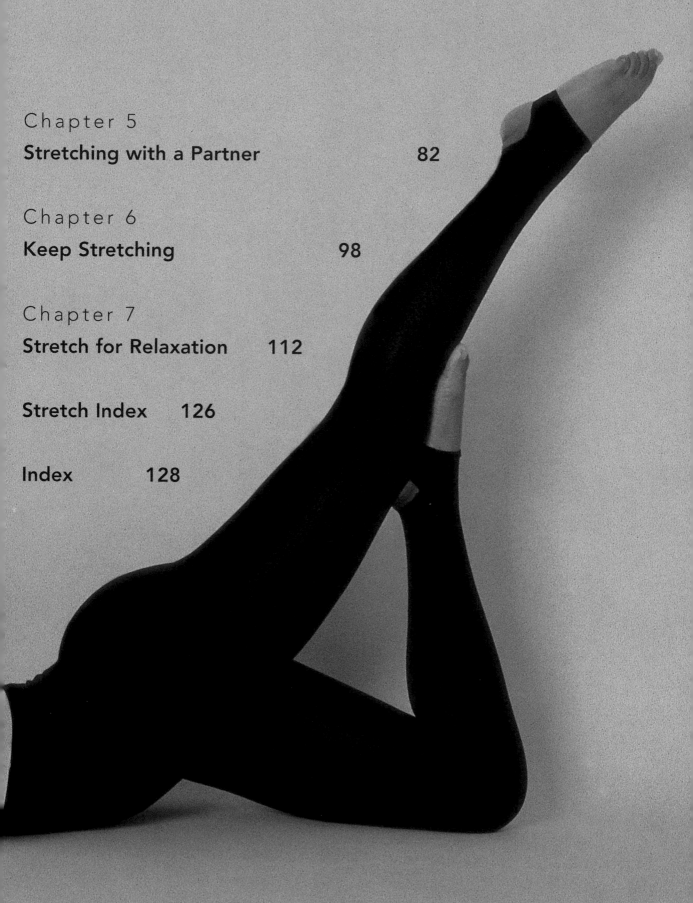

introduction

What I hope everyone will do with this book is flick through it to grasp a general idea of the contents, read through it to increase your understanding of the subject – and then use it!

This book is informative; there are easily understandable descriptions of all kinds of stretching methods and specially choreographed photographs to inspire the reader. Above all, this is a practical manual that can help toward greater flexibility.

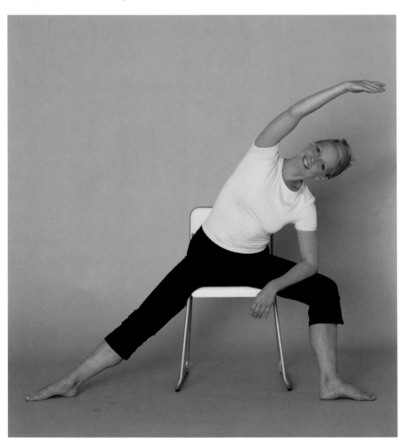

PRACTICE MAKES YOU "FLEXIBLE"

Like all physical pursuits, stretching requires practice. If you don't make the moves then you won't reap the benefits – so don't be tempted to just read this book like a novel and then put it down. You've got to get up and start putting it to the test! Try out the methods suggested to see which ones work for you and appreciate how good it feels to be moving and stretching those limbs!

You can start this book as a beginner or an experienced athlete – and whether stretching is a new concept to you or not, you will be enthused and informed by the explanations of stretch and the ways in which it can fit in as part of your daily routine and enhance different areas of your life. Did you know, for instance, that stretch can influence your posture and body image as much as it can improve your sporting chances?

In the first chapter you will find a definition of stretch and explanations that will clear up some of the misconceptions about stretching. This chapter will also give you plenty of reasons to improve your flexibility, both physiologically and mentally! Warm-up and mobility work is also covered, as these are essential components of any good stretch programme.

TRY AND TEST EVERYTHING

This book also provides you with a variety of methods for stretching. Some will increase your maximum flexibility and some will simply make you feel good. Either way there are chapters devoted to different stretching methods such as the PNF method, relaxation stretching and stretching with a partner – try them all and see which suits you best.

This book also provides you with a means of testing yourself and assessing your own flexibility level. Chapters 2 and 3 will help you to find your own level, your own shortcomings, and help you to set your own goals. With this information you can then use the beginner's, intermediate or advanced level programmes, which allow you to mix and match and progress to the next level as your flexibility increases. Don't forget to practise regularly though…

WARM UP AND COOL DOWN

If you have an interest in any sport at all, you will find some useful information in Chapter 4, which provides a comprehensive guide to the kind of stretches you should be doing prior to and after any major sporting activity. These stretches are specifically designed with a range of different sports in mind and they will help to loosen the right muscles and enhance your sporting abilities. Many sports are covered, from Football to Skiing and Cycling to Golf. There are also some key stretches and mobilizers, which should form part of all your pre- and post-sport stretch routines. Use this chapter as often as possible so that you memorize your stretches and can use them anytime or anywhere.

Hopefully, this book should be an inspiration to have some fun with your body! Take delight in feeling your body become more flexible and ready to move. Look at Chapter 5 for some ideas on how to work with a partner, or Chapter 6 for ways of getting yourself back to regular fitness and some unusual stretch ideas! There are stretches for problem areas and for relaxation purposes in Chapter 7. You can see already how many different ways stretch can be used.

ON THE MOVE

At the very end of the book you will find some moving stretch routines that are designed to be done to the music of your choice and as a means of self-expression or relaxation. Learn these and you will begin to learn by heart all the other stretches in the book – you will never be short of ideas to move and keep supple.

I wish you fun and flexibility, but remember – keep this book accessible and ready for action. Don't leave it on your bookshelf – get down on the floor and use it!

Chrissie Gallagher-Mundy

CHAPTER 1
introducing
stretch

The wonderful thing about stretching is that it can be so many different things to so many different people. It can provide a great starting point for getting your body into shape, an excellent all-round fitness programme, or the perfect complement to all kinds of sports and exercise regimes. However you choose to use it, you will no doubt discover that this is one of the most enjoyable forms of movement and exercise – and the perfect way to energize both the body and the mind.

A SENSE OF STYLE

Stretch forms a basic element of every major type of physical activity. This is especially true of activities where a certain physical "style" is important, where the shapes, movements, rhythms and dynamics that it is possible to express with the human body really come into their own.

The reason for this is that, unlike other elements of fitness, such as endurance-, stamina- or strength-building, stretch will begin to help you become physically and mentally aware of the shapes that you can create with your body. Stretch does this by giving you an instinctive feel for the way in which your body is aligned – how various parts, especially the shoulder girdle, ribcage, pelvis and limbs, should naturally be placed.

HAPPY MEMORIES

Once you understand a little more about stretching, you will find that it reminds you of whole areas of your body that you may have completely forgotten about over the years. For example, you will rediscover certain muscles that, once properly toned, can be used to lift and elongate the spine. This will help ease a whole range of posture-based problems, such as a painful back and aching joints. Stretching will also remind you of what it feels like to use your body as a tool, just as dancers do, allowing it to carry out all the instructions that your mind is giving it, easily and without stress.

A CO-ORDINATED APPROACH

Stretch also challenges your powers of co-ordination and simply shows you how good it can feel to move freely. You will soon be enjoying the forms and lines that you can create with your body simply for their own sake – time at last to stop worrying about the precise shape of your figure or how many press-ups you can do! Now you can begin to take pleasure in the sheer joy of dance and movement.

FIRST PRINCIPLES

Who should stretch? The answer is simple – everyone. Throughout this book, you will find programmes suited to people of all ages and abilities. It is, however, always a good idea to seek medical advice if you have any doubts at all about your fitness, or have any specific problems or injuries.

In this first chapter you will discover just what increased flexibility can do for you, in all kinds of different ways. You will also learn the all-important distinction between warming up and getting yourself moving fully – essential knowledge for anyone wanting a strong, supple body, one that is free from injuries, aches and pains.

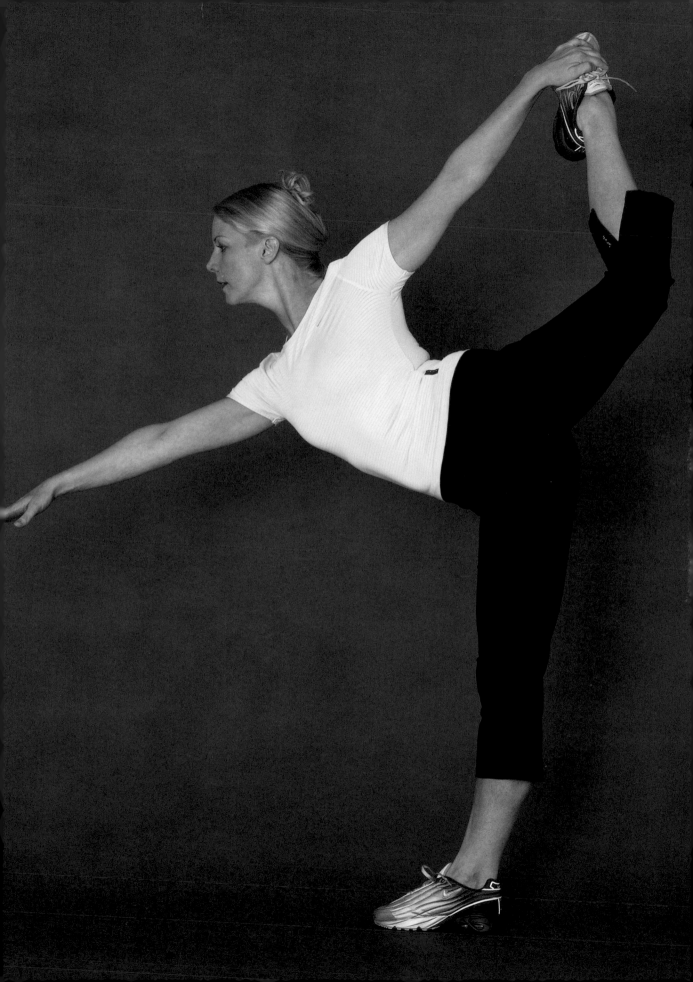

what is
stretch?

Before going any further, the whole idea of stretch needs to be defined properly, especially as there are various common misconceptions about the subject. Normally stretching means elongating the muscles of the body. The muscles, tendons, ligaments and joint capsules of the body all stretch to varying degrees and this in turn can give an impression of the whole body feeling elongated, extended and lifted.

TONING VERSUS STRETCHING

It is important to realize that stretching is not the same thing as toning. Toning involves contracting the muscles – usually against some kind of resistance – in order to extend or bend a limb.

This process challenges muscles, and with practice they will respond by developing greater tone – that is, becoming stronger and more shapely. Remember that, if you want to increase muscle strength, there has to be a degree of "overload" – working the muscle until it tires and fails, so that it responds by growing stronger. For example, most people have fairly well-toned biceps, at the front of the arm, because they are constantly working these muscles against resistance by picking up heavy objects.

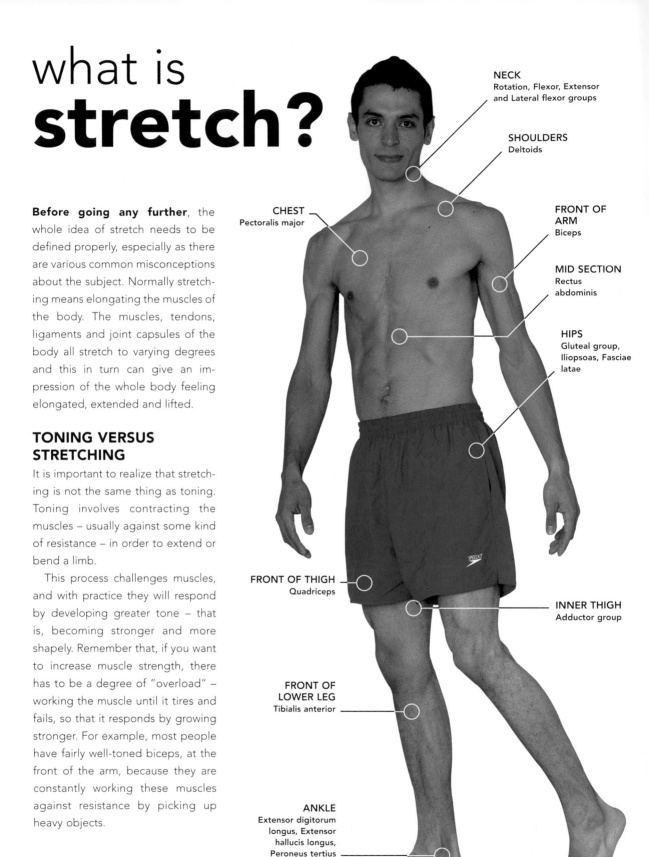

NECK
Rotation, Flexor, Extensor and Lateral flexor groups

SHOULDERS
Deltoids

CHEST
Pectoralis major

FRONT OF ARM
Biceps

MID SECTION
Rectus abdominis

HIPS
Gluteal group, Iliopsoas, Fasciae latae

FRONT OF THIGH
Quadriceps

INNER THIGH
Adductor group

FRONT OF LOWER LEG
Tibialis anterior

ANKLE
Extensor digitorum longus, Extensor hallucis longus, Peroneus tertius

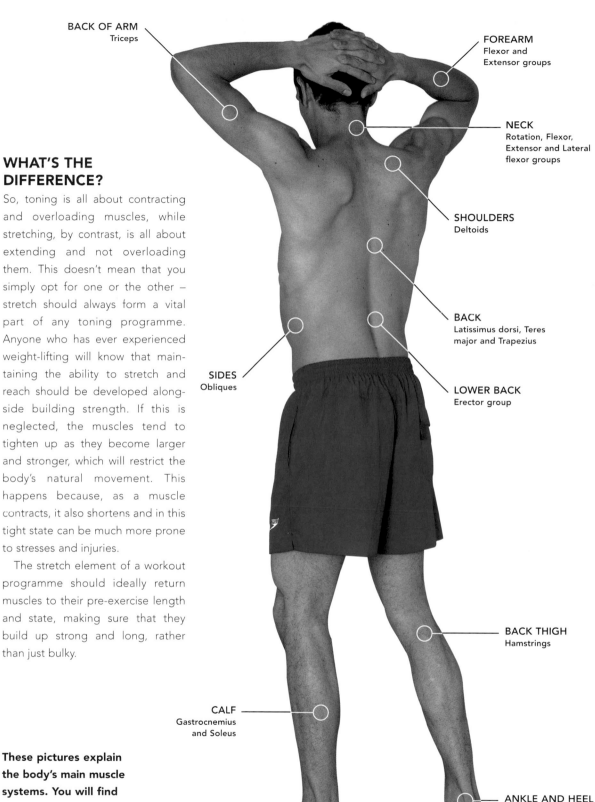

BACK OF ARM
Triceps

FOREARM
Flexor and
Extensor groups

NECK
Rotation, Flexor,
Extensor and Lateral
flexor groups

SHOULDERS
Deltoids

BACK
Latissimus dorsi, Teres
major and Trapezius

SIDES
Obliques

LOWER BACK
Erector group

BACK THIGH
Hamstrings

CALF
Gastrocnemius
and Soleus

ANKLE AND HEEL
Achilles tendon

WHAT'S THE DIFFERENCE?

So, toning is all about contracting and overloading muscles, while stretching, by contrast, is all about extending and not overloading them. This doesn't mean that you simply opt for one or the other – stretch should always form a vital part of any toning programme. Anyone who has ever experienced weight-lifting will know that maintaining the ability to stretch and reach should be developed alongside building strength. If this is neglected, the muscles tend to tighten up as they become larger and stronger, which will restrict the body's natural movement. This happens because, as a muscle contracts, it also shortens and in this tight state can be much more prone to stresses and injuries.

The stretch element of a workout programme should ideally return muscles to their pre-exercise length and state, making sure that they build up strong and long, rather than just bulky.

These pictures explain the body's main muscle systems. You will find these useful to refer back to as you go through the book.

body and
soul

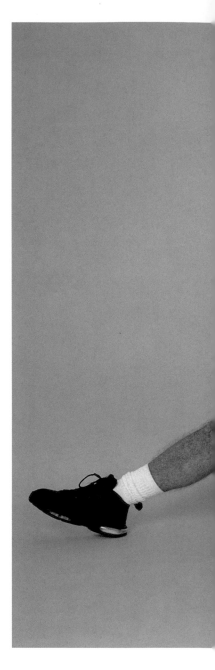

There are also types of fitness programme aimed specifically at developing endurance and stamina. These usually involve some form of aerobic exercise, which is designed to increase the body's uptake of oxygen. Aerobic programmes place extra demands on the muscles – especially the major muscles of the limbs, the heart and lungs – as the body learns to utilize the oxygen more efficiently. If prolonged, this type of exercise also draws energy from the body's fat reserves. Running, climbing and swimming are all good examples of popular endurance activities.

A STRONG BACK-UP

Stretching has no main part to play as part of an endurance activity, but it should always be used to provide a strong back-up. When muscles are worked hard, they need looking after and soothing. Stretch sessions can give your muscles a vital rest-and-recovery period, helping to de-stress and relax them. And because stretching makes your muscles more pliant and flexible, there is much less risk of any injury or pain resulting.

TAKING UP THE CHALLENGE

Although you can begin to see how stretching is a crucial component of various different types of health regimes, don't lose sight of the fact that it is a challenge in its own right – and a challenge that can transform different areas of your life. Improving your flexibility so that all your movements become much easier should not only be an intrinsic part of any sport or workout programme, but should also become a part of your everyday life.

ANCIENT WISDOM

The benefits of stretch, for both the body and the mind, have been appreciated for thousands of years, and it is this double reward that make it so special. Many ancient forms of meditation and exercise, such as Yoga and certain Martial Arts, rely heavily on the body's ability to push the boundaries of suppleness back even further while maintaining a focus on both control and strength. There is no shortage of good physical and psychological reasons for you to take up stretch – and once you start, you are sure to think of a few more!

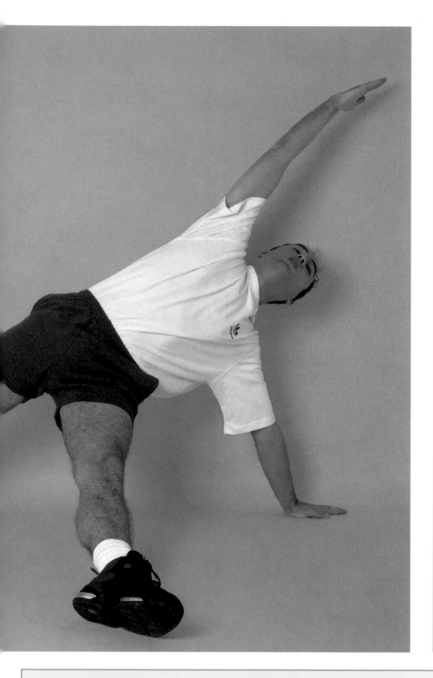

A HEALTHY MIND

Psychologically, stretch will:
- *Make you feel aware of your real self by putting you in touch with all of your body.*
- *Lead you to discover the "whole" you by revealing the vital links that exist between mind and body.*
- *Put you at ease with your own body by improving your range of motion and co-ordination. As you start to move and look better, so your sense of well-being will flourish.*
- *Provide a form of exercise and relaxation that is non-competitive and easy to do, meaning that motivation should seldom be a problem.*
- *Refresh your mind just as it energizes your body.*
- *Provide an oasis amid life's stresses and strains, helping you to deal with them more effectively.*
- *Ease your mind and body out of the various postures and positions that are causing all that mental and physical stiffness.*
- *Feed your creativity – create various shapes as you stretch and imagine yourself dancing, boxing, riding a horse; develop your fantasy life!*
- *Provide a pleasure that can be for you alone.*

A HEALTHY BODY

Physically, stretch will:
- *Return your muscles to their pre-exercised state and length.*
- *Allow you a full range of movement, without restrictions.*
- *Maintain this range of movement and so guard against aches and pains in the years to come.*
- *Provide a warm-up for further types of exercise.*
- *Provide a calm, wind-down session at the end of a workout.*
- *Keep muscles and joints mobile and flexible, and so reduce the risk of injury during exercise.*
- *Improve your posture and physical alignment.*
- *Improve the ease and quality of your movement.*
- *Help to ensure a healthy back – many physiotherapists prescribe it!*
- *Help you to relax and unwind, relieving muscle tension.*
- *Awaken muscles you never knew you had.*
- *Provide you with a way of exercising that you can do almost anywhere and anytime, with friends or alone!*

towards total **flexibility**

Stretching is all about extending the body and its muscular framework; discovering your level and seeing if you can improve it. Have a go at some of the following simple exercises:

- Next time you are reaching upwards, downwards or across, try gently stretching just that little bit further – it's always possible if you make the effort.
- Make yourself aware of movements that you find hard to perform quickly without feeling a strain. For example, sit in a chair and try reaching down towards the ground as if a pencil has rolled under your legs.

How does it feel? Or try standing at the foot of some stairs, with your hands firmly on the bannister, and place one foot on the first or second step. Now use your upper foot to lever yourself up. How high you go to start with obviously depends on the depth of the steps, but you should feel some stretch in your leg muscles. If you have no problems, try placing your upper foot on a higher step. Go gently and slowly, testing your body to see how much flexibility you have, and don't do more than you feel absolutely comfortable with.

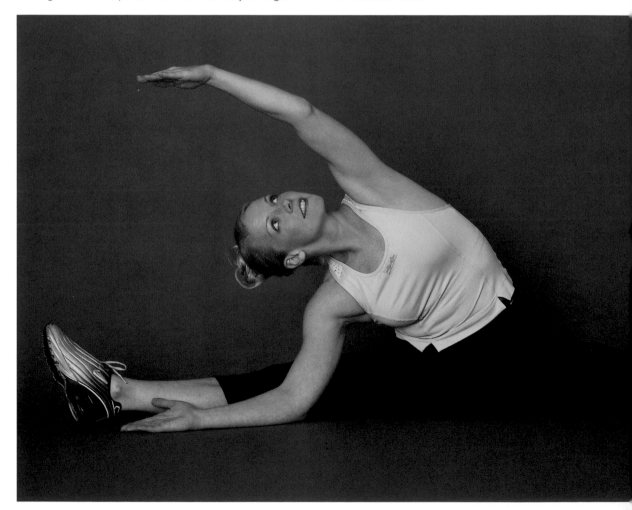

YOUR PERSONAL STRETCH PLAN

These kinds of exercises will give you some indication of just how elastic your muscles really are, and help to pinpoint the restrictions that you might want to improve. Our bodies are excellent at making adjustments, and if you keep repeating certain movements over and over again, your muscles will start to respond and will learn to stretch further and further.

The best approach is to follow a personally planned pattern of exercises, aimed at stretching specific muscle groups. Use the Stretch Challenge in Chapter 2 to help you identify the areas that need work and to plan a programme of exercises and goals that is tailored to your level of ability and needs.

STAYING MOBILE

To gain true flexibility, you need to use a combination of stretching and mobilizing. Mobilizing the body is not exactly the same as pure stretching, although it is closely allied. The emphasis is on movement in the joints rather than mostly in the muscles, and examples of good mobility would include:

- twisting around to see a passenger sitting in the back seat of your car without feeling any twinges or discomfort
- circling your arm past your ear painlessly and easily
- turning your head from side to side without feeling any "clicking" or pain.

Exercises aimed at improving mobility adopt a slightly different approach to stretching ones. They tend to consist of active movements, performed smoothly and consistently, whereas a stretch exercise involves assuming a position and holding it for a while to let the muscle elongate.

Mobility work will help to ensure that the synovial fluid that acts as a natural lubricant between joints is moving smoothly over the cartilage-covered, bony surfaces.

MOVING WITH EASE

Once the body becomes used to moving comfortably in a certain direction, the easier that movement becomes.

What happens all too often in everyday life is that we tend to get stuck in a rut of moving in very set types of pattern, repeating only a small range of movements that do not challenge all of our muscles. This means that certain muscles waste away, losing their strength and elasticity, and the mind-to-muscle co-ordination starts to slip. So, when we try to perform an action out of the ordinary – ouch! Suddenly there are twinges and stiffness where there should not be any.

Keeping the body moving in all the directions it can is vital. Your body is rather like a metal puppet, which needs to be kept well oiled in order to maintain smooth and unhindered movement that can be carried out just when, where and how you want it. With a carefully balanced programme of stretch and mobility exercises, this is just what you can achieve.

warming
up

The kinds of mobilizing movements just described are best used as part of a warm-up routine. Warming up the body before any prolonged exercise is one of the most important elements to concentrate on if you want to move without injury. Take your warm-up at a calm pace, using gently rhythmic turning and rotating movements in order to get the body accustomed to moving. You should be moving the joints slowly through their natural ranges of movement, as the joints' cartilage surfaces become accustomed to moving over each other smoothly.

You may notice a few "clicks" and "pops" at the start of your warm-up (sometimes due to trapped gases between surfaces). As you continue, the synovial fluid works to lubricate the joint surfaces and you will find that the creaks and clicks start to disappear and the movement becomes much smoother.

GETTING WARMER

The warm-up tells the rest of the body to get ready to move, and as everything gets into gear, you will gradually build up body heat. This increase in body temperature helps the muscles to become more pliable and supple, increasing the mechanical efficiency of your working muscles so that the contractions are more rapid and forceful. In other words, you are getting in touch with all those areas of your body that you may want to work effortlessly for you later on, so this warm-up puts you in touch – and in control!

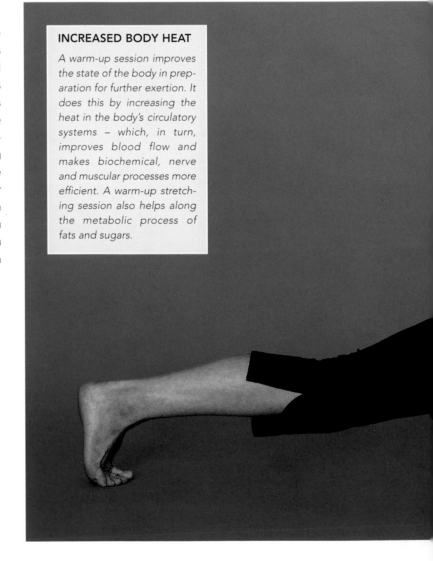

INCREASED BODY HEAT

A warm-up session improves the state of the body in preparation for further exertion. It does this by increasing the heat in the body's circulatory systems – which, in turn, improves blood flow and makes biochemical, nerve and muscular processes more efficient. A warm-up stretching session also helps along the metabolic process of fats and sugars.

THE JOINTS OF THE BODY

Our bodies have many different types of joint, with varying ranges of movement. Some are fibrous – bone connected to bone by fibrous tissue – while cartilaginous joints are connected by cartilage. Many of these joints only allow slight movement, or none at all. The joints that allow the greatest freedom of movement are known as synovial joints. In these, the end of each bone entering the joint is protected by cartilage and the joint cavity is lined with what is called a synovial membrane. This membrane secretes a nutrient-rich natural lubricant called synovial fluid.

The main synovial joint types are:

1 *Ball and Socket*
   Allows movement in all directions – e.g. hip and shoulder
2 *Hinge*
   Movement of a flex-and-extend nature – e.g. elbow
3 *Pivot*
   Rotation only – e.g. head
4 *Saddle*
   All movement except rotation – e.g. thumb
5 *Ellipsoid*
   Reduced ball and socket movement; virtually no rotation – e.g. knee and wrist
6 *Gliding*
   Two surfaces gliding across each other – e.g. joints between the vertebrae that make up the spine.

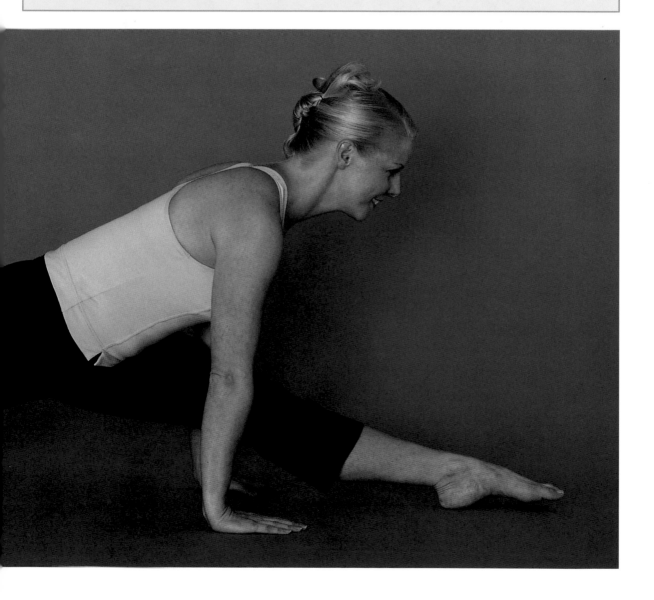

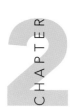

CHAPTER 2 finding your **level**

In this chapter you will find:

- A brief description of the various methods of stretching. There are different approaches available and some will suit you better than others. Some methods are also more appropriate at different times of the day or even at different stages in your life. There are more detailed explanations in the following chapters which will help you to understand a little more about the complexities of stretching and give you a chance to try the different methods safely.

- There is also a posture check which will teach you the correct starting position for all your stretch work. It will also help improve your general shape and stance and show you how to keep "lifted".

- A comprehensive flexibility test – the Stretch Challenge. This has been specifically designed to help you find your personal stretch level and to help you identify areas of your body where you may find that you are stiffer than others. Once you are more aware of your strengths and weaknesses you can use this as part of your tools for putting together a programme that works on the exact areas you need as an individual.

FIRST THINGS FIRST

Always go into moves slowly and cautiously, so that you and your body learn that stretch is a disciplined thing, and not something beyond your control or painful in any way. When you first begin, you may find even the mildest reach uncomfortable, but don't despair – it will simply be that your body is not used to the sensation of stretching. After a few sessions, you will soon find yourself getting used to the sensation, learning about your body and its limitations, and will feel more comfortable taking the stretch just that little bit further.

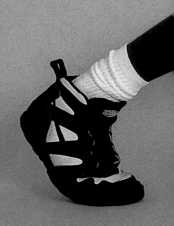

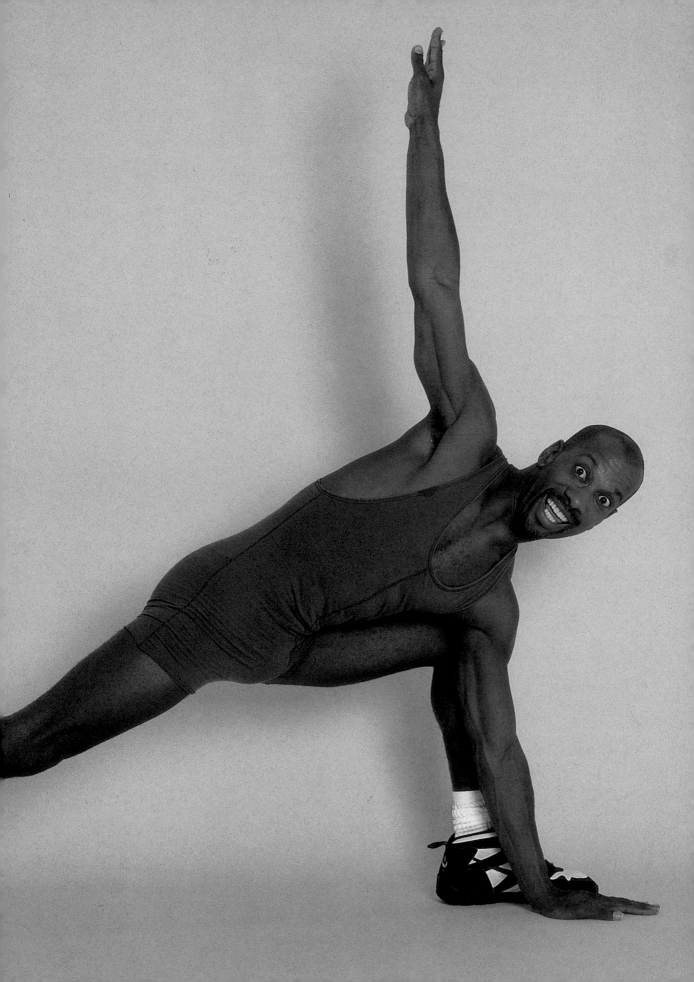

getting used to
the stretch

THE BASIC STRETCH

The main aim of stretching is to lengthen and extend the muscles a little further than they would naturally extend by themselves. Either before or after physical exertion, it is always a good idea to lengthen the muscles and to feel the body reach and twist, so that you rid yourself of any tightness that may have built up in the joints.

Stretching should feel pleasant, and not painful. The best general approach for a basic stretch is as follows:

- Find a comfortable stretch position that you can get into easily and hold without losing your balance. Try sitting with your legs apart and stretched out in front of you and then reach forwards, between your legs. This seated position is particularly good for beginners because your body weight is well supported and you will not be destabilized as you start to lean forwards. Also, the way your body weight is distributed tends to help the actual stretch.
- As you get into this stretch, you will feel some resistance in certain muscles (see The Stretch Reflex, page 22). When you feel this, just stay exactly as you are and simply register the tightness. Do not push yourself any further or come out of position. You should be feeling mild tension – just enough to tell your brain that certain

muscles are beginning to feel that they are being worked. You should not feel any pain. If this does happen, then return to an upright position and try again.

- After holding the stretch for 10–15 seconds, come out of it and return to your original sitting position. Now rest for 30 seconds, while gently moving the part of the body that you have just stretched – for example, in a seated stretch with legs astride, release the inner thigh muscles by slowly moving the legs in and out.

THE DEVELOPMENTAL STRETCH

This really means what it says: developing and holding the stretch a little longer so that the muscles lengthen even further. Follow these steps for the best results:

- Once again, take a comfortable seated position and start to lean in to your stretch until you feel mild tension and resistance.
- Hold the position until your body becomes accustomed to it – and keep breathing normally throughout the time.
- After about 15–20 seconds, the tension in your body should start to lift slightly and you will probably feel that you can lean a little further over. Don't push yourself; simply let your body weight ease you further over as you feel the muscle begin to lose some of its resistance.

The developmental stretch is really just a way of letting your body become used to the stretching sensation so that you can progress a little more, extending your stretch potential without discomfort or fear of injury. There are also various other ways that you can help your body to accept the stretch and extend it. For example, you will probably find it helpful to think about something other than the stretch while you are in position – your muscle will often complete its extension more comfortably and easily if the brain is distracted briefly and the muscle just allowed to "release" naturally.

NOW TRY THIS

Try this developmental hamstring stretch, which can be approached in two different ways:

1. BREATHE IT IN

- Lie on your back and hug one knee into your chest, really feeling the stretch in the groin area as you do so.
- Grasp your ankle and straighten your leg out as much as you can. Hold this position briefly, feeling the tension at the back of the leg, but only pull as far as you are able to without causing yourself any discomfort.
- Now breathe in slowly and, as you breathe out, pull the leg slightly closer to your face. It doesn't have to move a long way – just a few millimetres will do.

- Hold the position and repeat the breathing, pulling the leg closer still. Repeat this 3 times and you will be surprised at how much closer your leg is!

2. ROTATE AND STRETCH

Repeat as above, but instead of breathing in and out before you pull the leg in, get hold of the leg and simply rotate your foot first one way, and then the other. Now pull the leg further towards you. Repeat 3 times and notice how much further you are stretching your leg each time.

What both of these techniques illustrate is how the body and brain needs a little time to let the muscle achieve greater stretch. Also, this kind of stretching has a cumulative effect. If you repeat either of the above hamstring routines every day for just one week, and then do no exercise for two days (to allow the muscles to recover) and try the routines again, you will discover that your hamstring muscles will feel much looser than ever before.

And you can keep this feeling going – if you stick to a regular stretch programme.

TAKING IT FURTHER

Here are some of the other principal ways in which you can develop your stretching abilities:

1. BALLISTIC STRETCHING

This stretch involves small bouncing movements that push the body further into its stretch. It is often looked on as highly controversial, because injury is a little more of a threat with this approach. However, ballistic stretching can be effective if it is carried out carefully, especially as a preparation for activities such as dance and martial arts – the gentle, pushing movements of the body aid further stretchiness and help to prepare the body for more explosive actions. See pages 80–81 for more details on this method.

2. PNF STRETCHING

This stands for Proprioceptive Neuro-muscular Facilitation and is really just another way of "fooling" those muscles into relaxing a little more! If you contract a muscle strongly against a force for 10–20 seconds, its tone drops briefly immediately afterwards. If a stretch is applied at this point, you will achieve particularly good results. For more detailed directions on this technique, see page 85.

3. PARTNER STRETCHING

Stretching in company is an enjoyable way to pursue your stretch goals. You can work with anyone who is a similar size to you, even if your flexibility levels are different. What you must ensure is that you are both concentrating and working seriously to help each other.

The idea of working with a partner is to allow that person to use his or her strength to guide you into a deeper stretch – gently. If someone applies their extra body weight to yours, this can help to ease you into a more comfortable position, and sustained pressure will help the muscles to stretch further. There must, however, be lots of verbal and tactile communication between you so that everything is clearly understood and you stay within agreed limits. Specific routines and advice can be found on pages 82–97.

4. RELAXATION STRETCHING

Stretching for relaxation may seem like a contradiction in terms, but the two actually complement each other. Gentle stretching of stiff or tired muscles can be very relaxing to both the mind and the body – just the thing to revitalize and refresh you after a hard day's work! Although stretching and mobilizing are active pursuits, there are ways of assuming certain stretches that allow you to rest in those positions, letting your mind wander as your body really starts to relax.

Rather than being designed to develop greater flexibility, relaxation stretches are more to do with becoming fully at ease with the movement you already have. For details of the many different stretches that you can relax into, and for other ways to relax a tired body, turn to Chapter 7.

developing your **stretch**

One of the first steps towards developing your stretch technique is to improve your breathing, which will:
- calm you down
- help you maintain your stretches
- increase your stretching potential.

When you adopt a stretch position, don't hold your breath. Keep breathing normally, and check that you are doing this if you feel any muscular tightness. Holding your breath could increase your blood pressure, and it will certainly increase tension and discomfort.

DEVELOPING YOUR FLEXIBILITY

We all start out with pretty good flexibility – it's only through misuse or lack of use of certain areas of the body that we stiffen up. Once you are following your own programme regularly, you should find stretching a pleasurable, relaxing thing to do and will start to become aware of your physical limits.

To increase your flexibility, you may want to include some developmental stretching – where you stay in a position a little longer to allow a specific muscle to stretch that little bit further. As before, always start with a warm-up session, and bear in mind how some of the body's basic reflexes work.

THE STRETCH REFLEX

When a muscle is stretched, it soon starts to send messages to the brain to tighten that muscle and halt the stretch, especially if it was sudden. This reaction is known as the stretch reflex. It is activated by a muscle's change in length and by the speed of the movement and is necessary not only to protect the body against overstretching, but also to maintain muscular control during normal postures such as standing or sitting.

AUTOGENIC INHIBITION

There is, however, another reflex that acts in opposition to the stretch reflex and this is known as autogenic inhibition. As the tension in stretching muscles increases, this event is registered by special organs found in the body's tendons (which attach the muscles to the skeleton). These organs send signals to the brain, telling the muscles to relax and preventing the stretch reflex from occurring. This autogenic inhibition reaction also stops muscles from contracting so hard that they pull away from the bone.

> ### BREATHE DEEPLY
>
> *To take a comfortable stretch position further, concentrate on breathing in slowly and deeply through the nose and then releasing the breath slowly through the mouth. Breathing acts as a good distraction technique when a stretch needs to be prolonged, making you concentrate on your breathing rather than on how your muscles are feeling. As you come out of the stretch position, keep your breathing even and regular in order to prevent you from snapping out of a pose and possibly causing an injury.*

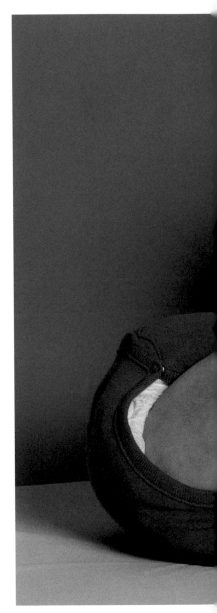

PUTTING IT ALL TOGETHER

These two reflexes do not occur at the same time, and everyday movement is unlikely to trigger autogenic inhibition. Both reflexes, however, do have an effect on how we should stretch. Rapid or jerky stretches, for example, simply activate the stretch reflex and tighten the muscles, whereas smooth, sustained (at 30 seconds or longer) stretching of warm muscles allows them to relax

and the stretch reflex to become desensitized. With developmental stretching, autogenic relaxation will occur, overriding the stretch reflex.

The best way to perform a stretch is in a stable, comfortable position where some part of your body weight can assist you. For example, if the hamstring muscle of your right leg (see pages 10–11) is already quite supple, but you want to develop it further, a good position might be to sit with your legs open

and straight out to each side and your body leaning over your right leg. You can then perform the stretch slowly and gently, holding this position for 10–20 seconds. You might then be able to hold it for 30 seconds or more, letting the weight of your upper torso take you further as the muscles become less resistant. This kind of stretching starts to develop your flexibility because it allows the muscles to relax gradually – and perfectly safely.

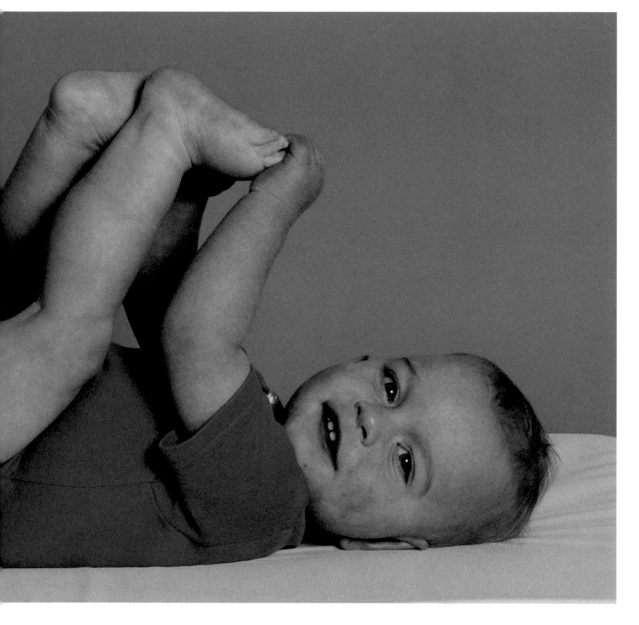

perfecting your **posture**

Toning and lengthening your muscles not only leaves you feeling refreshed and revitalized but is also very important for good posture.

- In all areas of the body, it is important that muscles are pliable and flexible to avoid problematic aches and pains – particularly if there are inflexibilities on one side of the body rather than on the other. A stretching programme can really help to even up irregularities in the body – and also keep your stance correct and relaxed.

- To support the body in its natural alignment, you need stomach and back muscles that are strong but also flexible – not tight and bunched up. If the lower back muscles are very tight, and particularly if the stomach muscles are also weak, then the arch of the lower back may become too exaggerated. This, in turn, tends to make the ribcage bow outwards, throwing the body weight back over the heels so that the bulk of the upper torso's weight rests on the lower back. This can cause back problems, as well as unattractive posture.

UNEVEN STRESSES

Similarly, if the buttock or hamstrings are very tight, the lumbar curve can be pulled too straight, causing uneven stresses and problems in the back and legs. Try lifting one leg off the ground, while keeping it fairly straight. Is this easy or can you feel tension and a pull on the pelvis, making it tuck underneath you? This feeling can be extremely restrictive and destabilizing. (If you do feel a tightness here, turn to the stretch index on pages 126–127.)

PULL YOURSELF TOGETHER

Whenever you are sitting or standing in one place for any length of time, try to remember to pull up through the torso and the spine. Make sure your head is not arched back or collapsed forwards and that your stomach muscles are working and supporting the spine so that there is no pressure on the lower back.

Next, check for any major tensions that you might be feeling. The most common places for tension are the lower back, the back of the pelvis and across the shoulders. As well as noting the tension and seeking to release it by visualizing its release (see opposite page), this will also give you an idea of the areas you may want to stretch out later. For instance, if you have been hunched over a desk for a long time, it is always a good idea to take the body in the opposite direction – arch backwards to relieve the muscles.

GENTLE BACK STRETCH

Try this relaxing back stretch.

- *Lie on your back with your arms stretched out to the side, your legs bent and your feet flat on the floor.*
- *Now slowly lower your knees all the way over to one side and rest there.*
- *In this gentle twist position, you will feel the lower back release and the stomach muscles start to relax. You can now concentrate on slowly feeling all the muscles in your arms relax so that your shoulders sink towards the floor.*
- *There should be no stress in the neck or shoulders. One knee is resting on the other, so the legs are free of tension and the lower back is "opened up" slightly. If you were to rock the knees from side to side, resting for 10 seconds on each side, this would mobilize the back while providing a very relaxing and pleasurable exercise.*

REDRESSING THE BALANCE

To attain a good, postural stance, follow this routine.

- *Stand with your back to a wall, and with your heels touching that wall.*

- *Pull in on the stomach muscles and tilt the hip bones up toward you to help push your lower back closer to the wall. Check that the ribcage is pulled up, and has not sunk on to the hips. The shoulders should be relaxed, not held up or forced back. Drop the chin slightly to ensure that the top of the spine is straightened.*

- *Now take one step away from the wall and try to relax your body slightly. Stand there for a little longer and then start to embark on a mental journey through your body. Think first about your shoulders and about the muscles across the back of your neck and your upper back (see also pages 10–11). Picture the muscles lengthening and widening, even though you are not actually making any physical adjustments. Simply imagine the tensions being released in this area and the muscles expanding in response.*

- *Now picture a line running from the very tip of your head right down to the soles of your feet. As you stand there, this line is lengthening your spine – lifting the top of your head nearer to the ceiling while pressing your heels firmly into the floor. Don't make any physical adjustments, simply allow the illusion to release tensions and let the muscles learn how to extend and relax.*

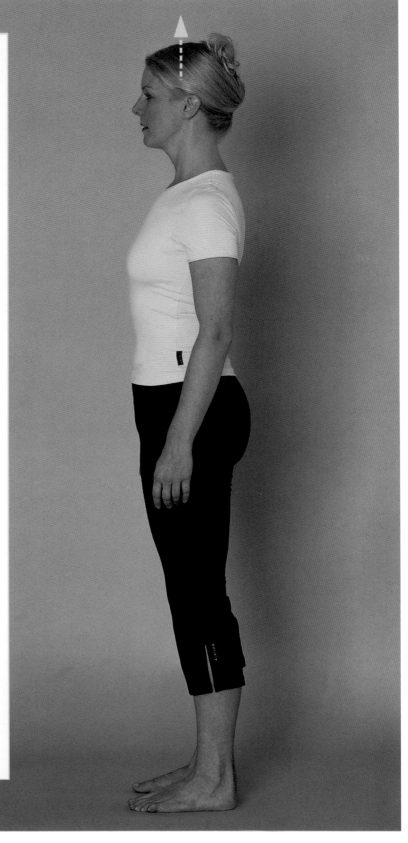

the stretch
challenge

The four exercises featured on pages 28–31 are designed to let you assess your stretch capabilities so that you can then go on to devise your personal stretch programme in Chapter 3. They are effective ways to warm up your muscles for activity. Once you work through them and are feeling properly warmed up, you are then ready to take the stretch test.

Start with Exercise One (page 28), which is relatively simple, and work your way through to Exercise Four, on page 31. For each exercise, start out by attempting the Beginner's position, which has been colour-coded with a pink background. Look at the photograph and attempt to get into a stretch that is as close to this as possible. However, do not force anything and if you feel any part of your body threatening to cramp, come out of the position and "shake yourself out" before re-attempting it. When you are in the position, you should be able to feel a stretch, but no pain. You should also be able to hold this position for at least a few seconds while breathing normally and without feeling too much strain.

Between each stretch, you might want to shake yourself out and "jig" around gently before attempting the next position.

PRE-ASSESSMENT WARM-UP

Before you try to assess your flexibility, you should give yourself a little warm-up. We can all stretch better when our bodies are warm and you want to know what you are really capable of, so give yourself the best possible chance!

- *March up and down on the spot for about 3–4 minutes and then continue to march but now reach your arms first upwards and then downwards at the same time.*
- *Bend your knees and squat down, with your thighs no lower than parallel to the floor, and then reach up as high as you can. Repeat several times.*
- *Swing your arms across your body so that you twist first one way, then the other. Make sure only your upper body twists.*
- *Finally, go into a light, on-the-spot jog for 3 minutes until you feel your body warm up nicely. While you are jogging, make sure that, as your foot hits the ground, contact goes from the toes to the ball of the foot and through to the heel. This will help to absorb any shock far more effectively.*

MOVING ON

If you feel fully comfortable with the Beginner's position, then you might like to attempt the Intermediate position, always shown with a yellow background. Perhaps you find this quite easy, in which case move on to the Advanced position, with its blue background. Always remember – don't push yourself.

SCORING

As you go along, you should be keeping score for each exercise. Once you have found a position that reaches your limits, give yourself marks as to how comfortable and manageable that position really feels. For example, if you are happy with the Beginner's position and don't feel that you want to push this particular exercise any further, then

HOW TO SCORE	
BEGINNER:	1–3
INTERMEDIATE:	4–7
ADVANCED:	8–10

mark yourself between 1 and 3, depending on how comfortable the position is to you. If you are happier at the Intermediate level, then give yourself a mark between 4 and 7, and so on, as shown above. What you should end up with is one score for each exercise.

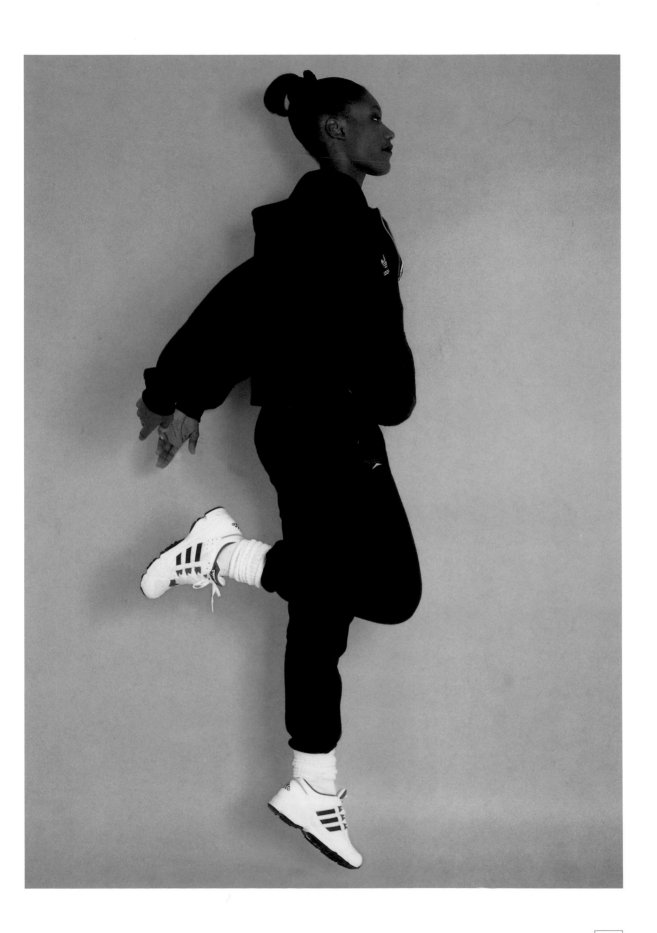

COMBINATION STRETCHING

You need to bear in mind when trying these four exercises that they are all combination stretches. This means that they do not focus on stretching just one muscle, but they can involve many muscle groups in different parts of the body. Because this is what is involved in most everyday activity and sports moves, combination stretches are the best way to test yourself.

You may find that one part of the stretch is easier than another – this is because you are perhaps more flexible in one area than another. For the purposes of this test however, judge the stretch as a whole when you are deciding how comfortable and manageable it is.

Now look at the boxes entitled 'What You Might Feel' to further personalize your programme. Decide which category shown – from beginner, intermediate or advanced – describes you. This will help you to alter your programme so that in areas where you have slightly more flexibility (or less) you can take things a little further.

EXERCISE ONE:
WHAT YOU MIGHT FEEL

- *BEGINNER'S position:
  a stretch in the groin area.*

- *INTERMEDIATE position:
  this requires some flexibility
  in the torso.*

- *ADVANCED position:
  this also needs flexibility in
  the torso, and it also increases
  the groin stretch.*

BEGINNER'S POSITION

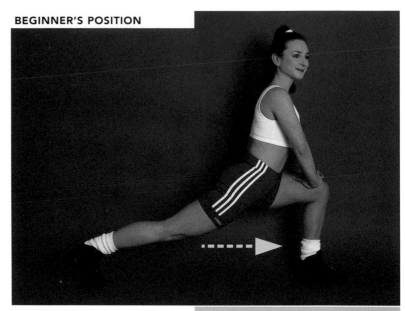

INTERMEDIATE POSITION

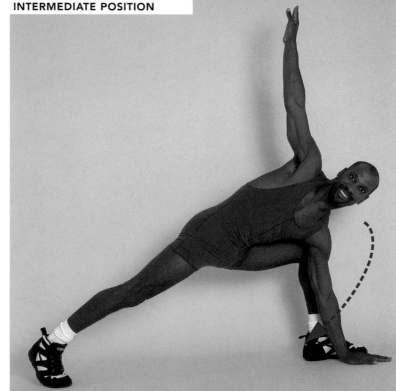

ADVANCED POSITION

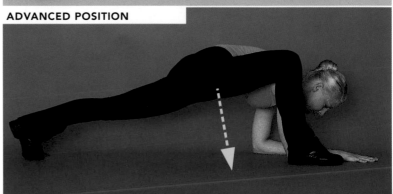

BEGINNER'S POSITION

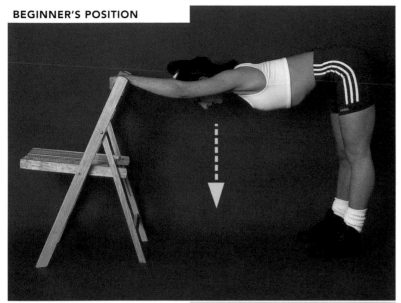

INTERMEDIATE POSITION

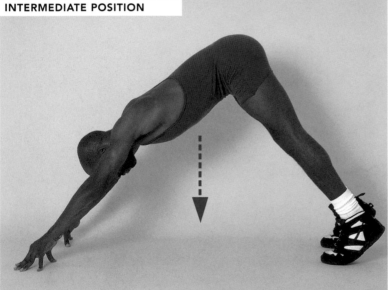

ADVANCED POSITION

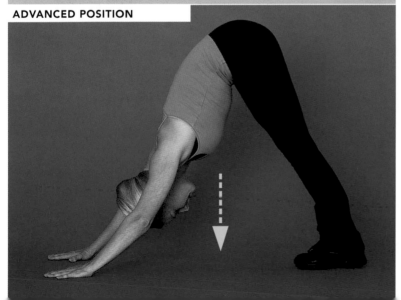

EXERCISE TWO: WHAT YOU MIGHT FEEL

- *BEGINNER'S position:*
  a stretch up the back of the legs and in the shoulder area.

- *INTERMEDIATE position:*
  you might feel an additional pull up the back of the calves.

- *ADVANCED position:*
  you should feel extra tension in the back of the legs and some flexibility in the back.

BEGINNER'S POSITION

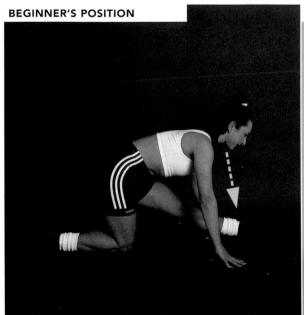

INTERMEDIATE POSITION

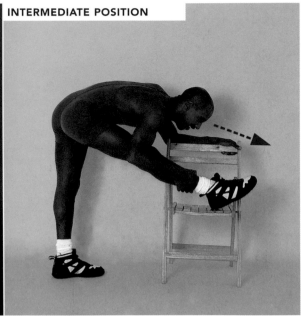

ADVANCED POSITION

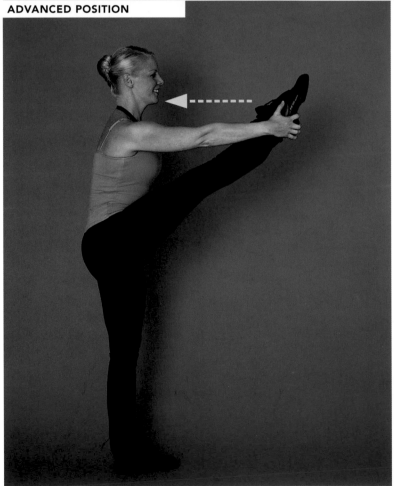

ASSESSING THE TEST RESULTS

Once you have completed all the four exercises, give your body a gentle, all-over shake and then march up and down on the spot, lightly, to release the muscles from their sustained positions. After any stretch session, including this one, make sure that you keep warm and rehydrate – so replace any clothes you may have discarded and drink a large glass of water before you sit down and look at your scores.

EXERCISE THREE: WHAT YOU MIGHT FEEL

- *BEGINNER'S and INTERMEDIATE positions: a stretch at the back of the legs and, depending on your flexibility, a stretch in the lower back area.*

- *ADVANCED position: same as above, plus additional flexibility in the groin.*

BEGINNER'S POSITION

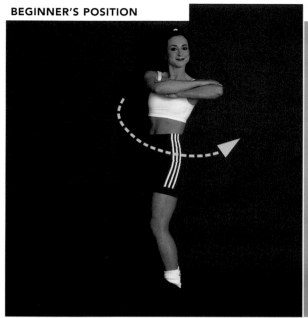

INTERMEDIATE POSITION

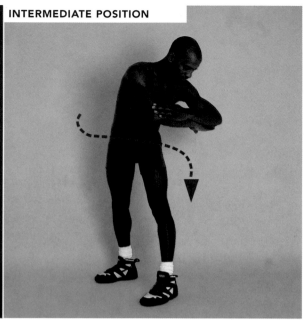

You should now have a score for each of the four exercises. Add these scores together to give yourself one overall total and turn to pages 32–33 to discover which level of programme this score qualifies you for and how you can tailor it to your own personal needs. Next, turn to Chapter 3 to follow your programme to find a stretchier you! Keep a note of what you scored on each individual test, as this will be used to add to your basic stretch programme. When you have worked out your programme, it doesn't matter at what level you start – you will undoubtedly improve with time! Once you familiarize yourself with the exercises for your level and practise them regularly, you will probably find that you can reach the next level very quickly. To judge what progress you have made, simply redo the stretch challenge.

ADVANCED POSITION

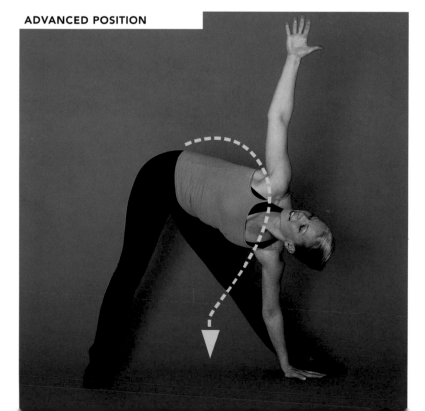

EXERCISE FOUR: WHAT YOU MIGHT FEEL

- *BEGINNER'S position: a stretch around the torso and back.*

- *INTERMEDIATE and ADVANCED positions: an additional stretch in the back of the legs and hips.*

setting your **level**

Having worked through the exercises on the last four pages, you will now have an overall score. This tells you which basic level you belong to.

YOUR SCORE...

A total score of 4–12:
BEGINNER'S LEVEL

A total score of 13–30:
INTERMEDIATE LEVEL

A total score of 31–40:
ADVANCED LEVEL

Now you have identified your level, turn to Chapter 3 and study the stretch programme for that level.

Now look at the boxes on the right to further personalize your stretch programme. Assess your level according to the statements in the boxes; this will help you to alter your programme so that in areas where you have slightly more flexibility (or less) you can take things a little further. This will ensure that your body is being stretched as far as it can in all directions while keeping things safe as you progress. Don't forget to pursue your stretch programme regularly so that you notice ongoing improvements and benefit from them.

If you found any of the Beginner positions very uncomfortable or difficult:

* Stay with your BEGINNER'S programme and work through it regularly. As you keep working on it, you will develop more stretchiness and if you go back to the Stretch Challenge exercises (pages 28–31) some weeks later, you may find that all the positions have become a lot easier.

If you managed Intermediate level comfortably on Exercise 1:

* Add Position 4 of the INTERMEDIATE programme in Chapter 3 to your schedule.

If you managed Advanced level comfortably on Exercise 1:

* Add Position 4 of the ADVANCED programme in Chapter 3 to your schedule.

If you managed Intermediate level comfortably in Exercise 2:

* Add Position 1 of the INTERMEDIATE programme in Chapter 3 to your schedule.

If you managed Advanced level comfortably in Exercise 2:

* Add Position 4 of the ADVANCED programme in Chapter 3 to your schedule.

If you managed Intermediate level comfortably in Exercise 3:

* Add Positions 1A and B of the ADVANCED programme in Chapter 3 to your schedule.

If you managed Advanced level comfortably in Exercise 3:

* Add Position 2, 2A and 2B of the ADVANCED programme in Chapter 3 to your schedule.

If you managed Intermediate level comfortably on Exercise 4:

* Add Position 5 of the INTERMEDIATE programme in Chapter 3 to your schedule.

If you managed Advanced level comfortably in Exercise 4:

* Add Position 3 of the ADVANCED programme in Chapter 3 to your schedule.

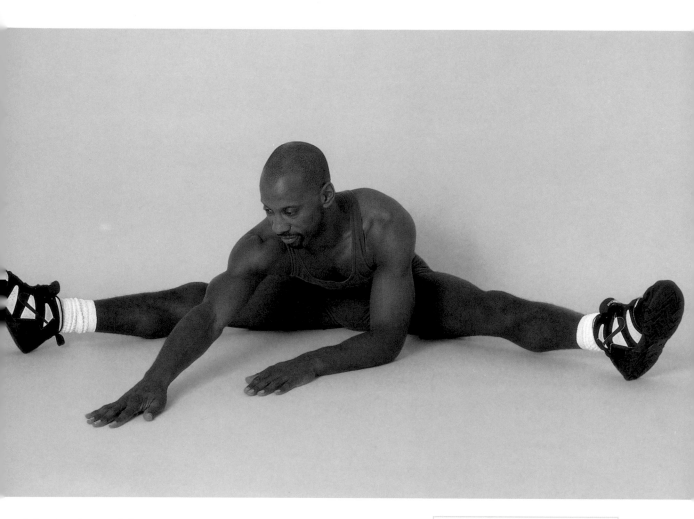

GETTING PERSONAL

To personalize your programme to an even greater degree, go back and look at your individual marks for each exercise. Use them to make the adjustments shown on the right to the programmes outlined in Chapter 3. These adjustments apply whether your basic level is Beginner, Intermediate or Advanced.

KEEPING NOTES

Make a note of all the exercises you should be adding to your programme. What you have now is a truly personal and challenging schedule which, if you follow it regularly, will develop your stretching abilities to the full.

You may find from attempting the tests that you identify an area of your body, such as the lower back or hamstrings, that is particularly stiff. Once you have made this useful observation, turn to Chapter 6 (and to the Index) to find the stretches that are relevant to your specific problem area.

SAFETY CHECK

If you feel excessive pain in any of the stretches you have just tried, a check-up with your local physiotherapist would be a good idea. The physiotherapist can double-check that there are no muscle or bone injuries, or other conditions, that may be affecting your ability to stretch.

3 CHAPTER your personal stretch **programme**

Now that you know which basic level is just right for you, here are the three stretch programmes: Beginner, Intermediate and Advanced. You should be following most of one of these programmes, perhaps with some exercises borrowed from the other two to personalize your stretch routine even further (see pages 32–33).

BEFORE YOU START

There are two important things to think about before turning to your personal programme:

1 Breathing – getting this right will help you to develop a really good technique (see page 22).

2 The "stretch reflex" – this gives you a greater understanding of how your body is reacting to the stretches (see page 22).

LISTEN TO YOUR BODY

As you stretch, concentrate on what you are feeling – listen to your body. You should feel an extending sensation in your limbs when you take up the positions, but you should not feel pain. If you move into a stretch too quickly, or push too far, you will activate the stretch reflex (see page 22), which is the body's way of automatically protecting itself from over-stretching by suddenly tightening the muscles in question. If you always feel comfortable when you are stretching, you won't push too far and so will avoid unnecessary injury.

TWO ALTERNATIVES

When you begin your programme, start slowly. Ease into the stretch and concentrate on listening to what your body is feeling. When you have held the position for the stated time, or for as long as it feels comfortable, come out of the stretch as slowly as you went into it and give your body a little shake. Then, if you want to, you can repeat the stretch once more. There are really two ways of developing your technique:

1 Ease into a position, hold it for the appropriate amount of time, and then release it slowly.

2 Ease into the stretch and then move around gently, perhaps rocking slowly in and out of the stretch, in order to get yourself used to the general feeling. You might find that this is a good way to become comfortable with a stretch that you have never tried before. Under no circumstances should you bounce, as this can traumatize or pull the muscles.

You must decide which of these methods – probably a combination of the two – works best for you.

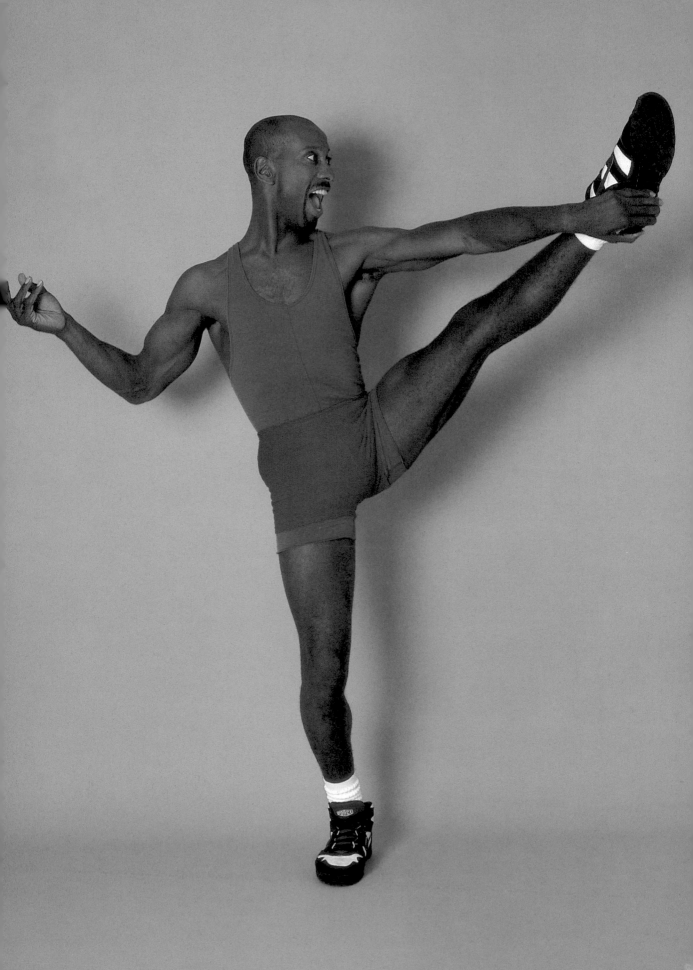

beginner's stretch
routine

When beginning your stretch routine, remember to find a warm, private room and start with a gentle warm-up. Make sure that your clothing allows you to move freely and try playing some inspiring music! You may want to use the annotated photographs on pages 10 and 11 to guide you around the different muscles.

POSITION 1:
STORK STRETCH

- You might need to hold onto the wall or some other immovable object to help you balance as you reach behind to grasp your foot.
- Position the bent knee in line with the straight knee and pull the foot gently towards the buttock.
- You should feel a stretch along the front of the leg – this exercise is principally stretching the quadriceps muscles in the front of the thigh.
- If you feel a pull in the knee-cap, you may need to release the stretch a little.
- To increase the stretch, pull in on the stomach muscles and tilt the hips up and in, towards you.
- To include a groin stretch, start to tip your body forwards so that the bent leg and upper torso become parallel with the floor.
- Hold this position for 20–30 seconds, and then shake out your bent leg.
- Repeat twice on each leg.

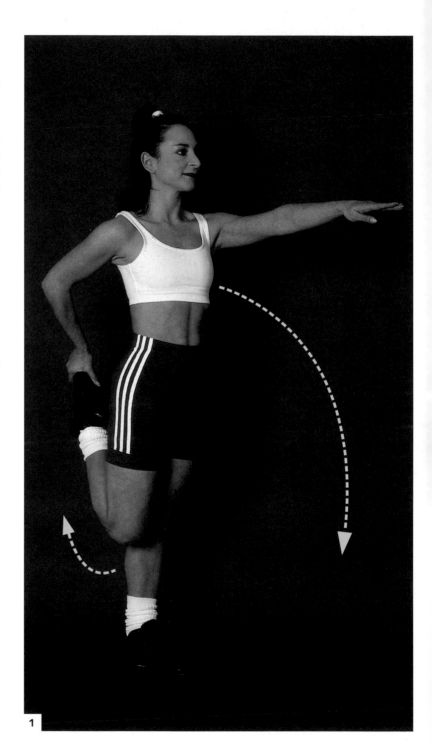

1

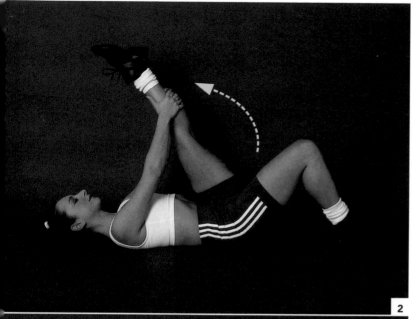

POSITION 2:
CLOCK HANDS

- Keeping the raised leg as straight as you possibly can manage, gently pull it towards your nose. If you can't keep your leg totally straight, don't worry – simply pull it in gently as far as you can without causing any discomfort.
- You will feel a stretch at the back of the leg – this exercise principally stretches the hamstrings found at the back of the thigh.
- Don't allow your hips to be pulled off the floor.
- To increase this stretch, breathe in slowly and, as you breathe out, pull the leg a little closer to you.
- Hold this stretch for 20–30 seconds and then relax the leg.
- Repeat twice on each leg.

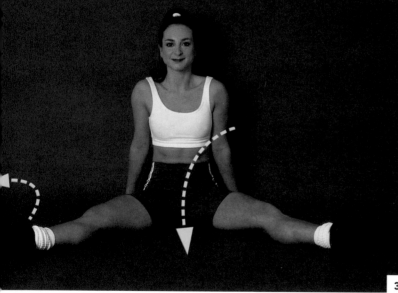

POSITION 3:
WIDE STRETCH

- If you find it difficult to sit with your legs apart while keeping the back straight, it may help to place your hands on the ground behind you to provide some additional support. Use the leverage of your hands to push your torso slightly forwards.
- If you have enough flexibility, place your hands on the floor in front of you; if this is too difficult, simply rotate your feet backwards as far as you can and release.
- You might feel this stretch in various places in your body, depending on where you are tightest. You may feel some stretch in the lower back, for example, the back of the legs or the inner thighs. This exercise principally stretches the adductors on the inner thighs.
- If you feel a harsh pull in the knee area, move your legs slightly closer together.
- Hold this position for 30 seconds.
- Repeat 3 times, but do a different exercise in between.

POSITION 4:
ARCHED STRIDE

- Make sure that you have the weight of your body pressed towards the front leg as you bend into your lunge, with your back toe acting as stabilizer. Now press your arms back behind your ears as far as you can.
- You will feel a stretch in the groin area as you hold your lunge, as well as a stretch in the shoulders. This exercise is stretching the adductor muscle group and the gracillis muscle on the inner thigh, and also the deltoids in the shoulders.
- Don't sink into the lunge, but keep the body lifted and ready to push out of the stretch.
- Hold for 20 seconds before shaking out.
- Repeat 3 times.

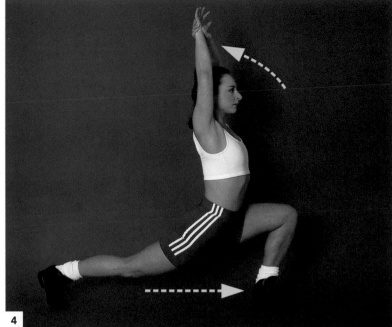

POSITION 5:
BACK BEAUTY

- If you have not done this stretch before, stand in front of a wall and use this as a support. Keep your torso fully lifted as you arch slightly backwards. Pull up in your abdominal muscles.
- You will feel a flexing in your lower back and a stretch in the abdominals.
- You should not feel any pain – if you do, come out of it and try again without leaning so far.
- As you become more confident, you can start to arch slightly further, as long as your hips stay stable and you have a wall behind to stop you from falling too far.
- Hold for just 15 seconds.
- Repeat twice.
- Recover by lifting up and then curling your upper torso forwards.

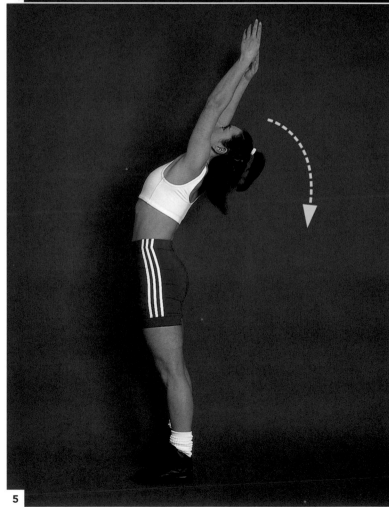

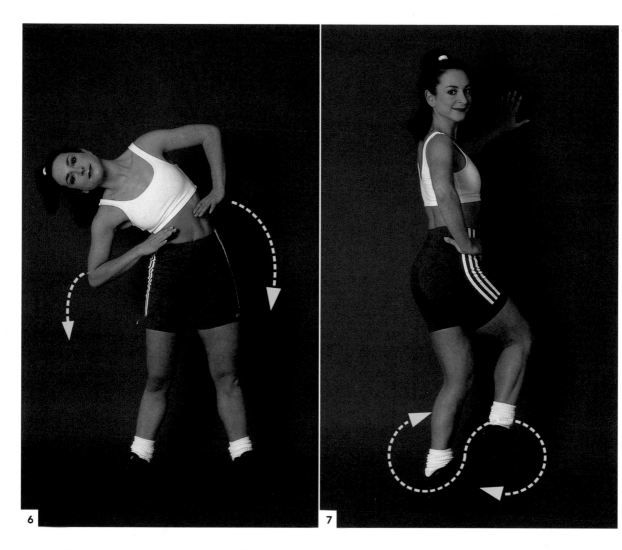

6

7

POSITION 6:
SIDE SWING MOBILIZER

- This is a mobilizing exercise (see page 15) so, as you move gently from side to side in this position, you should be keeping a steady rhythm going.
- You should feel the sides of your body being stretched and the length of the torso becoming more flexible as you move.
- Don't bend so far that the sides of your body feel wrenched, and don't drop your head too far over – you should keep it in line with your body.
- Swing from side to side up to the count of 20.

POSITION 7:
FIGURE 8 MOBILIZER

- Holding on for support, swing your bent outside leg around in a large figure 8 shape. First, your bent leg should swing forwards, across the front of your body, and then back in towards your other knee. It should then circle outwards, towards the back and around, so that your bent knee goes behind your straight leg, before coming back around to its starting position once more. Let your supporting leg bend a little as you perform the figure 8 mobilizer, and keep your abdominal area lifted.

- The hip joint of your bent leg should be turning right round, and this is where you should feel the movement. It should also become easier and smoother as it continues.
- Keep swinging for 30–40 seconds, really reaching all parts of the figure 8.
- Repeat 3 times on each leg.
- This will help to keep the hip joints flexible and creak-free.

intermediate
programme

Start with a gentle warm-up. Once warm, keep lots of layers on and don't stop moving during your workout. Try using music to dictate some different tempos for the exercises that have more movement in them.

POSITION 1: **STEP UP**

- Use a sturdy chair or stool to rest your foot on as you push your hips forwards.
- You will feel the stretch underneath the legs and groin, particularly the thigh of the leg on the floor – this stretch is for the adductors and hamstrings and the quadriceps.
- Hold the stretch for 15–20 seconds, shaking the legs out in between stretches.
- Repeat twice on each leg.

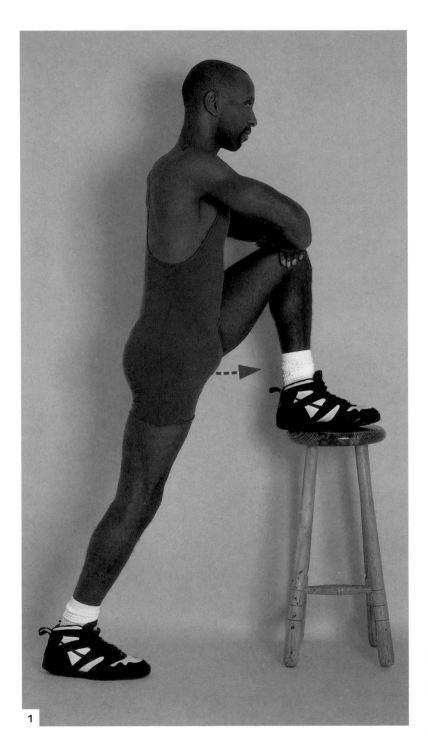

1

POSITION 2: **FLAT OUT**

- Start with your hands reaching high above your head and reach out as you start to bend over towards your leg. Try to keep your back as straight as possible as you lean over. When you can't go any further, rest your hands on your leg, above the knee.
- You will feel a stretch in the back of the raised leg and possibly also in the lower back. This stretch is mainly to elongate the hamstrings at the back of the thigh.
- Don't round or collapse the back and let the head hang. Instead, try to keep the back as straight as possible, with help from the abdominal muscles.
- If you can rest your hands easily on your thigh, then you could gradually try to get near enough to rest your head there as well.
- Hold for 30 seconds.
- Repeat 3 times with each leg.

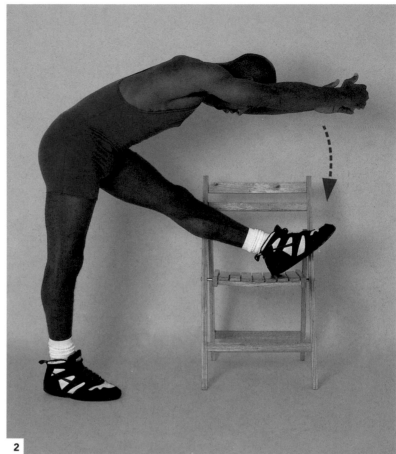

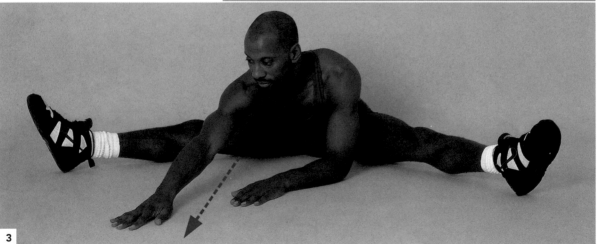

POSITION 3: **FORWARD CREEP**

- With your legs outstretched and apart, see how far forwards you can lean and begin creeping further forwards with your hands to extend your stretch.

- You will feel the stretch on the inside of the legs – this stretch is for the adductors.
- You should not feel too much of a pull on the knees or the back of the legs – if you do, creep back slightly.

- If you let the weight of your torso pull you forwards and bow your head, the stretch will increase.
- Hold for 30 seconds and then come back and gently massage your inner thighs.
- Repeat twice.

POSITION 4: **THE UPEND**

- Link your hands behind you before you tip your upper body forwards and push your arms towards the floor.
- Keep your knees just slightly bent and you will feel a stretch on the back of the legs as well as the underarms. This stretch will extend the hamstrings and to a certain extent the deltoid, pectoral, biceps, Teres major and tricep muscles surrounding the humerus (the bone of the upper arm).
- Hold the position for a count of 16 and then bend the knees as you come upright.
- Repeat twice.

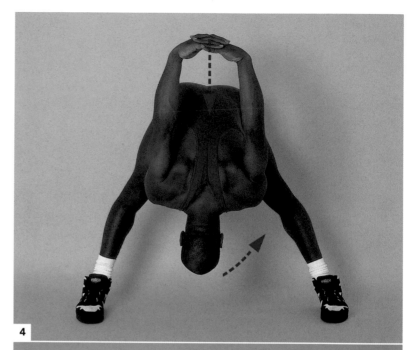

POSITION 5: **CURVACEOUS MOBILIZER**

- Reach up as high as you can before leaning over to one side, but don't stop there – continue to curve the arm around to the front so that the upper body is curved forwards before it rolls to an upright position.
- You should feel a pleasurable stretch in the upper back and side of the torso – this movement will stretch the trapezius and rhomboid major, which are the main muscles in the upper back.
- You can let the stretch involve more of the back if you curve further over as you come round to the front. Make sure, however, that you keep the abdominal muscles pulled up and stable.
- Repeat 5 times each side.

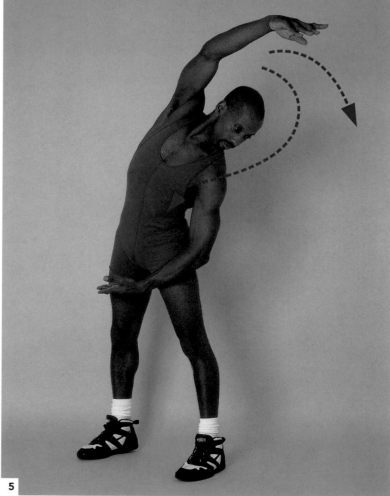

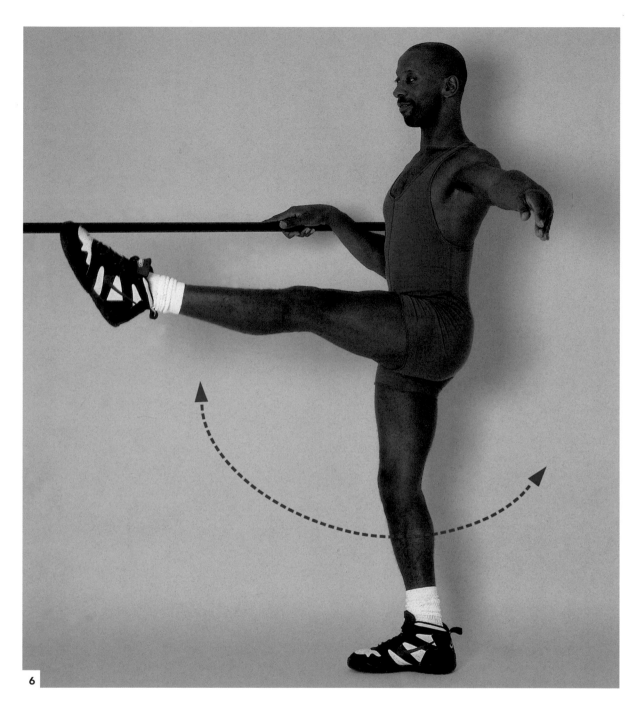

6

POSITION 6:
THE SWING MOBILIZER

- Always make sure that you are warmed up before commencing this mobilizer.
- Stand straight and tall, holding on to a bar for support, and gently swing your leg back and forth, at a low level.

- You will feel the leg starting to loosen in the hip and the front and back of the thigh starting to stretch slightly.
- Make sure that the swing is the same height at the back as it is to the front.
- Try to keep the knee of the supporting leg as straight as

you can and keep the hips still – do not let the pelvis be pulled underneath.
- Perform between 8 and 10 swings on each leg.

advanced
programme

Make sure that your body is warmed up and comfortable before you start your programme. Move into the positions carefully and try to make the transition from one pose to another as smooth as possible.

POSITION 1: **THE CRAB**

- Step backwards into a lunge, with the back leg straight, and lower your hips as close to the ground as possible. Make sure your front knee is positioned directly over your toe.
- Now swivel inwards a quarter of a turn so that your bent knee is out to the side of your body and your hands are reaching out in front.
- You will feel a stretch in the groin area and the inner thighs and some working of the mobility in the hips. This stretch combination mainly involves the adductor groups, the hamstrings, gluteals and quadriceps.
- Don't allow the bent knee to turn inwards once you are in the second pose and make sure the knee of the straight leg is facing the ceiling.
- If you want to increase the stretch, keep the heel of your bent leg flat on the floor.
- Move into the first position and hold for 15 seconds, then move into the second pose and hold for 10 seconds.
- Repeat by turning back into the first pose and repeating the sequence again.

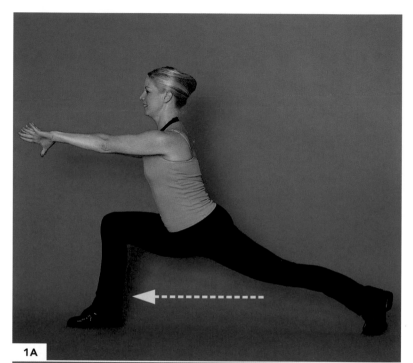

1A

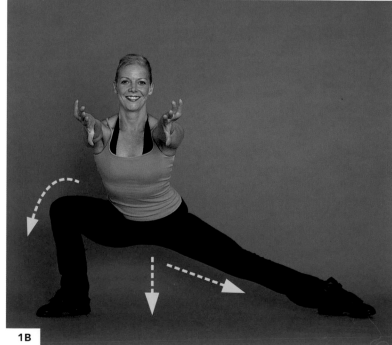

1B

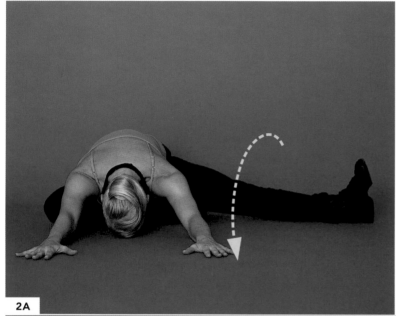

2A

POSITION 2:
WALKABOUT

- Sit as far forward as you can in the first pose shown (2a), keeping both buttocks touching the floor.
- Keep the back as flat as you can as you extend the arms forwards on to the floor.
- You will feel a stretch in the lower back as well as in the hip joint of the bent knee, and possibly on the inner thigh of the straight leg.
- Next, turn towards your extended leg and pull your chest towards your leg (2b). Breathe out as you press as far over as you can. Then gently release.

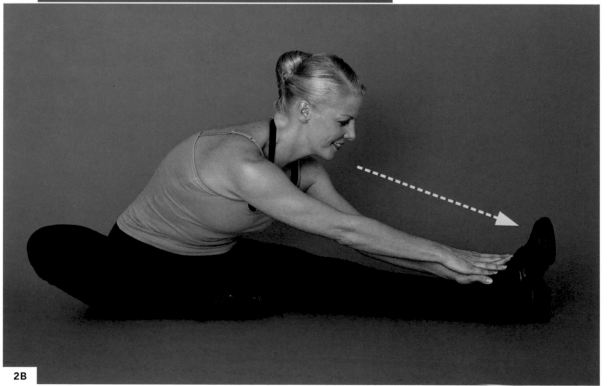

2B

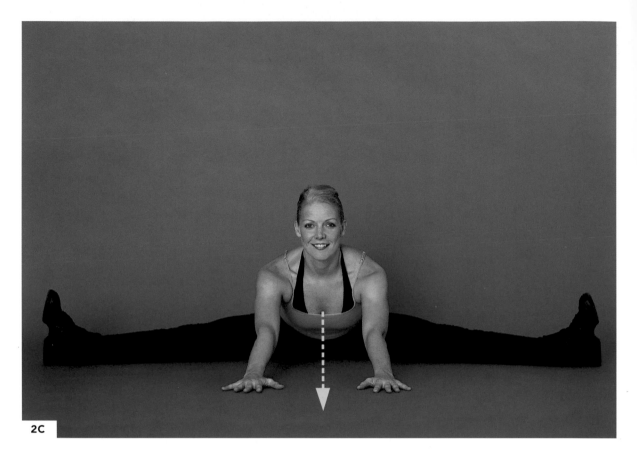

2C

POSITION 2: **WALKABOUT CONTINUED**

- Finally come back to the centre before extending your second leg. Now breathe in and as you breathe out press the chest and arms forwards, pushing the chest as near to the floor as your inner thighs will allow (2c). From 2a–2c you will feel a stretch in the sides of the legs (inner thighs and at times the outside thigh) and also in the sides of the torso and possibly the back. This will involve the adductor muscle groups, the hamstrings, the gluteals, the quadriceps, the oblique muscles of the abdomen and the Latissimus dorsi.
- You should feel a gentle pull in these areas – not pain.
- Hold each pose for 20–30 seconds and move smoothly into the next.

To recover, use your hands to push you up and your abdominals to help your back curl up gently to an upright position.
- Repeat this sequence twice on each leg.

POSITION 3: **ROTATING MOBILIZER**

- Pull up in the knees and keep the legs straight and the hips fixed as you rotate your upper torso around that axis. Start by rotating at a shallow angle and build up to a rotation position where the back is parallel with the floor at all times. This is a very advanced exercise, so it will take some practice to do.
- You will feel the upper torso mobilizing and every part of the torso being stretched. The exercise involves the oblique and rectus abdominal muscles and the Latissimus dorsi.
- Rotate once each way, return to an upright position, and breathe especially deeply.
- Repeat 3 times.

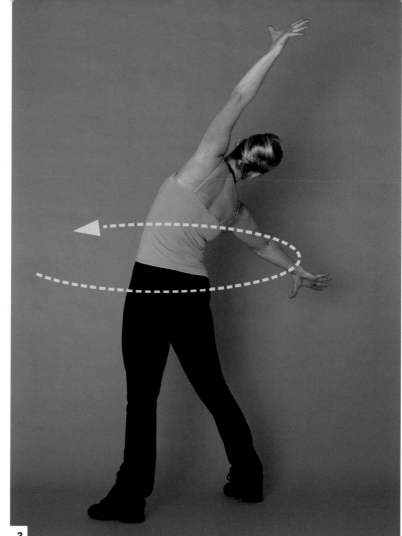

3

4

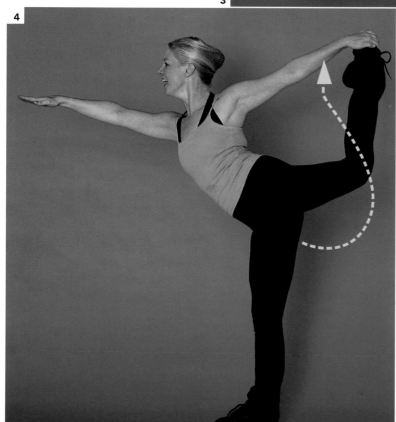

POSITION 4: **OLYMPIC STANCE**

- Holding on for balance if necessary, reach behind and hold onto the calf. Now, keeping the leg behind you, start to lift and straighten it as far as you can.
- This requires great flexibility in both the front and back of the legs, the groin area and the lower back. It involves the hamstrings, gluteals, quadriceps and the adductor muscle group.
- Raise the leg only as high as you can without losing balance and tipping forwards too far.
- Stretch into the position slowly.
- Try the position twice on each leg.

making stretch
a habit

If you have never tried a regular stretch programme before, you need to concentrate on developing good habits right from the beginning.

- Set a regular time aside for your routine. Allow yourself a small amount of time to begin with – 15–20 minutes is plenty – so that you are less likely to postpone the workout just because you haven't enough time.
- Find a comfortable place where you can avoid interruptions. Your chosen spot should be warm, draught-free and with enough space for you to stretch out in all directions.

> **MOVING TO MUSIC**
>
> *Try using different pieces of music to match your mood. In this way, you can make your routine a relaxing end-of-the-day stretch one day and a revitalizing pick-me-up the next!*

GETTING STARTED

When you are ready to start your stretch programme, place the book in front of you and make sure you have warm clothing on that won't restrict your movements. Start with a quick warm-up, by following the example on page 26 or by doing whatever it takes for you to feel warm and loose. A jog is a good way to warm the body and its muscles, as is a quick spell in a sauna or steam room, if you have access to one.

Whenever you stretch, make sure that you are fully concentrating. Turn the answerphone on so that you don't have to leap up quickly if someone calls – one of the easiest ways to pull a muscle! Begin the stretch in a comfortable, stable position and stay warm. A mirror may be useful, to check that you are in the correct position, but is not absolutely necessary. And always make sure that you can get out of the position before you get into it.

MOVING ON

As you continue with your stretching programme, your body will become more accustomed to the moves and you should find the stretches becoming smoother. You should also find yourself stretching farther, but always make sure that your hands (or other body parts) are there for support, so that there is no risk of slipping or lack of control.

Don't be too impatient for results and always stretch with caution. You should feel the stretch sensation in the belly of the muscle rather than at the extremes. If you feel too much of a pull at the joints, for instance the back of the knees, insides of elbows or deep in the lower back, then ease off slightly. With regular practice you will get to know your body and its warning signs – a correct stretch feels pleasurable rather than painful.

After a stretch session, you should feel revitalized, relaxed and perhaps a little hungry. The next day, you should feel no ill effects. If you are stiff or have aches and pains, then you could well have overdone it. You do not want to damage or tear your muscle fibres – so start GENTLY.

GETTING GOOD RESULTS

Stretching must be done regularly and correctly for it to make a real difference. If you do your stretch programme properly, there is no reason why you shouldn't practise a short session as frequently as every other day if you want to see some rapid results. A day's rest in between is always a good idea to let the muscles recover. The great thing is that elasticity in the muscles really can improve pretty quickly – you will be surprised at what you can achieve in as little as two weeks.

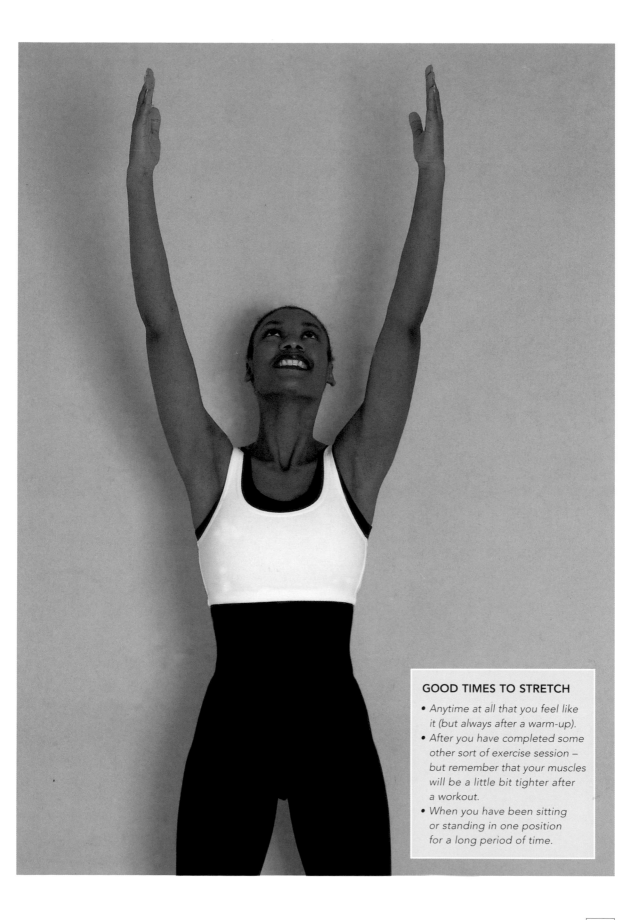

CHAPTER 4 sporting **chances**

Whatever sport you enjoy, there are stretches you can do that will help you to get even more out of your sporting activities. What you will find here are stretches specially designed to enhance warm-up and cool-down procedures for your chosen sport. As you will see from flicking through this chapter, every sport has its own specific stretches, and most activities also have some stretches in common.

Turn first to the core stretches and mobilizers illustrated and described on pages 53–57, and use these as part of your warm-up routine, to prepare your body for the exertion to follow. Now, turn to the stretches that are designed specifically for your sport and work your way through these. At the end of these stretches, you should be prepared for just about anything the game or activity can throw at you!

FLEXING YOUR SPORTING MUSCLES

Most sport activities utilize the large muscles of the body. These include the deltoids (shoulders) and the pectorals (the chest area) as well as the abdominals (the stomach area) and the major leg muscles: quadriceps, hamstrings and calf muscles; gastrocnemius and soleus. (Refer to pages 10–11, for a guide to the major muscles.)

WARM UP AND COOL DOWN

As we have already mentioned, stretching is not a substitute for a proper warming up procedure – however it is an important part of the warming-up and cooling-down process. When you begin whichever warm-up routine you use before your chosen sport activity, you should start by doing the moves that are aimed specifically at increasing your body temperature.

You should now start with the core stretches and core mobilizers outlined on the following pages. These will continue the warm-up process and help your body and mind to rehearse the kinds of moves you will be making in your sporting activity. This is why the stretches shown in this book are as close to actual sports moves as possible. If you can keep your stretches similar to the actual moves you may be making, then your body will be that much more prepared.

BEFORE...

Once you have performed your sports stretches, you are ready for your game, so, if you are not due to play immediately, wear something warm to keep the thermal effect going a little longer. If you get delayed enough for the muscles to start cooling down, then you may have to repeat a few more stretches just to get you moving again.

...AND AFTER

After your game, you will be hot and your muscles will be warm and "buzzing". This is not, however, always the best time to stretch out. Although your body is warm immediately after hard exercise, the muscles are tightened due to repeated contraction. Try to give yourself 10–15 minutes to re-adjust and cool down; just walk around slowly and let the muscles rest.

Once you feel rested, you can begin your cool-down stretches. Repeat some of the core stretches and mobilizers included in the section for each sport. Adopt the position and ease into it gently. You are aiming to gently extend the muscles to their pre-exercise length and rid them of any tension gained during exercise. While you are performing these stretches, you are giving yourself a mental and physical breathing space – perhaps to think about your game and the improvements you can make next time around.

Only stay in the stretch for as long as it feels comfortable; feel the muscles release instead of trying to develop the stretch. After a hard game is not the time to go for a developmental stretch.

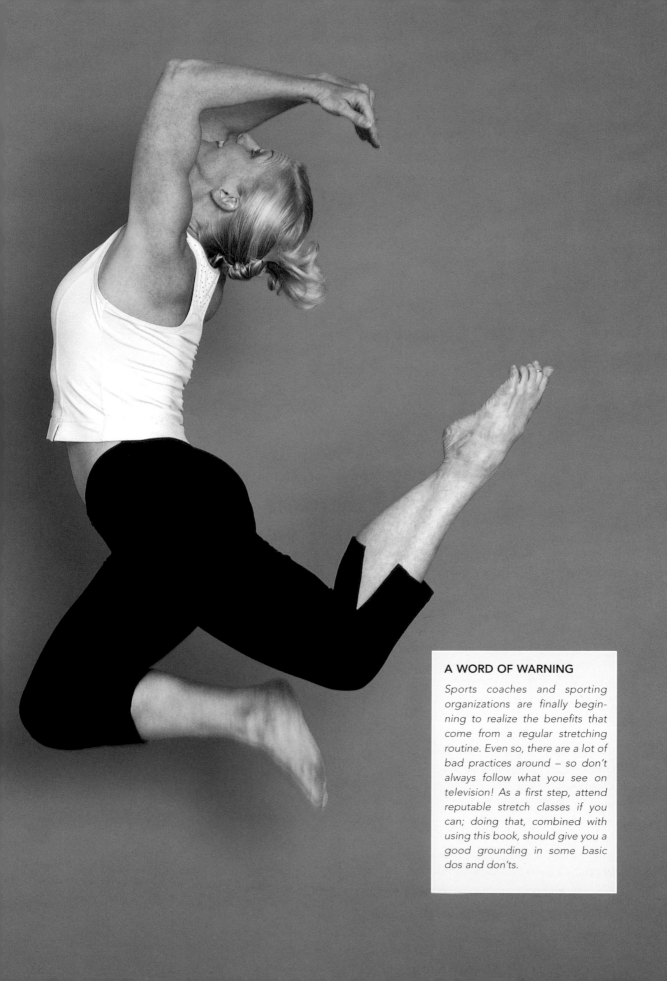

A WORD OF WARNING

Sports coaches and sporting organizations are finally beginning to realize the benefits that come from a regular stretching routine. Even so, there are a lot of bad practices around – so don't always follow what you see on television! As a first step, attend reputable stretch classes if you can; doing that, combined with using this book, should give you a good grounding in some basic dos and don'ts.

coping with
stiffness

Muscle stiffness can come in many forms, from the not so painful to the excruciating! It can range from the odd twinge in one muscle or another to an overall ache that might make you feel that you have a bad case of flu.

THE DEBATE CONTINUES

There is still a great deal of debate over what exactly causes muscle stiffness. One theory is that it is caused by over-worked or over-stressed muscle fibres sustaining microscopic tears. While these tears gradually repair themselves, the healing process produces general soreness. Other theories talk about muscle "ascemia" – a build-up of bodily chemicals, such as lactic acid, that could send the muscles into spasm and cause stiffness.

What is known for certain is that, as with most things that occur in the body, the reaction sets in at a later stage. This means that, with severe stiffness, the pain may actually come on one or two days after the strain has taken place and sometimes even increase during the third day. This is known as DOMS or Delayed Onset of Muscle Soreness.

WHAT CAN YOU DO?

Theories on the best way to deal with stiffness also differ, although it is generally accepted that very stiff muscles need time to recuperate. So, if you have been through a hard workout, it is best to spend the following day letting the body relax and the muscles recover. If you do feel soreness, then muscle rubs,

saunas or a hot bath can help relieve some of your aches. If the pain or stiffness is really troublesome, then Aspirin or Arnica (a natural healing agent) may help.

THE HAIR OF THE DOG

If you really have to be active on a day when you are very stiff, then the best way to deal with the aches and pains is to warm up thoroughly and then go carefully but firmly into some of the moves and stretches that you did the day before. If you work through the same moves that made you stiff, it will help to relieve your stiffness so that you can exercise with less pain.

If you have an actual injury such as a muscle tear, then pursuing your sport on the same day is probably not advisable and rest may be more appropriate. If in any doubt, rest up – or see a doctor.

WHEN DOES STIFFNESS STRIKE?

You may well experience stiffness if you have:

- played a particularly hard game
- made a move that your body wasn't used to
- not played your sport for a while.

AVOIDING STIFFNESS

Some tips on avoiding stiffness:

- *It is thought that reducing the amount of "eccentric contractions" – extending the limb against resistance – in your workout (for example, holding a 5 kilo dumbbell in bent arm position and extending the arm slowly twenty times) may help to prevent severe stiffness.*
- *If you train regularly, the body seems better able to adapt and severe stiffness reduces considerably.*
- *An adequate cool-down and stretch-out period reduces the risk of severe muscle stiffness.*
- *Heat and massage can help relax and rejuvenate tired muscles, flushing fresh blood through to the stiff areas, which then carries away potentially toxic – and thus stiffness-inducing – products.*
- *A hot shower immediately after exercise reduces stiffness more effectively than waiting until you get home to have a shower.*
- *The main cause of stiffness is people throwing themselves into routines they are unprepared for and being overenthusiastic during the first few sessions. Pace yourself, give your body time to adapt and save your boundless enthusiasm for regular, sustained training, not short, sharp bursts!*

core **stretches**

Use these basic stretches as part of your warm-up and cool-down routines, before and after your sporting session. These core stretches should be followed by the core mobilizers on pages 56–57 and then by the warming-up and cooling-down stretches designed specifically for your sport. You can also use the core positions as part of your warm-ups and cool-downs before and after any kind of fitness activity, such as a stretch session or aerobics workout. Whatever kind of stretch you are doing, it is important to remember that:

- your posture should be good, with your body properly aligned – follow the photographs carefully for this
- you are as relaxed as possible when you begin each move
- you should keep breathing normally throughout all your stretches.

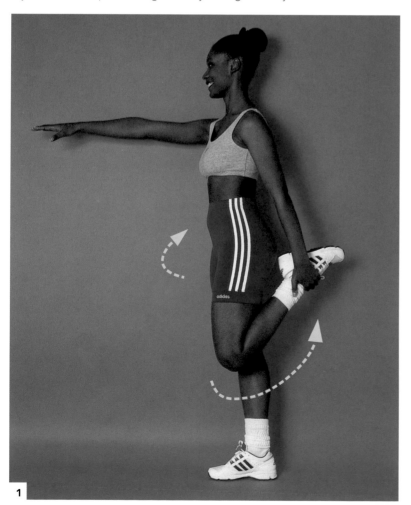

1

WATCH YOUR POSTURE

Many of the curling, bending or leaning movements may involve one part of the body without affecting others. However, there are plenty of movements that work several different areas, and bad posture in one will affect the others. During some of the more complicated stretches, you may be tempted to let your overall posture go as you try to increase your stretch, but you must always maintain the proper alignment of the body in order to stretch the correct muscles and avoid the risk of injury.
NB: "Workout" refers to any form of exercise or sporting session.

POSITION 1: **THIGH STRETCH**

- Extending your arm will help you balance in this position.
- You should feel a stretch sensation in the front of the thigh.
- To increase this stretch, check that both knees are level, pull in on the stomach and tuck the hips up and under, towards you.

Before Your Workout: Hold for 20 seconds.
After Your Workout: Hold for 30 seconds.

POSITION 2: **BASIC LUNGE**

- Once you have mastered this basic stretch, it will lead you into many other stretch combinations.
- You should feel a stretch in the groin area and in the back of your calf.
- The lower you go in this position, the more you will increase the stretch, but make sure you don't lose your balance.

Before Your Workout: Hold for 20 seconds.
After Your Workout: Hold this stretch for 25 seconds.

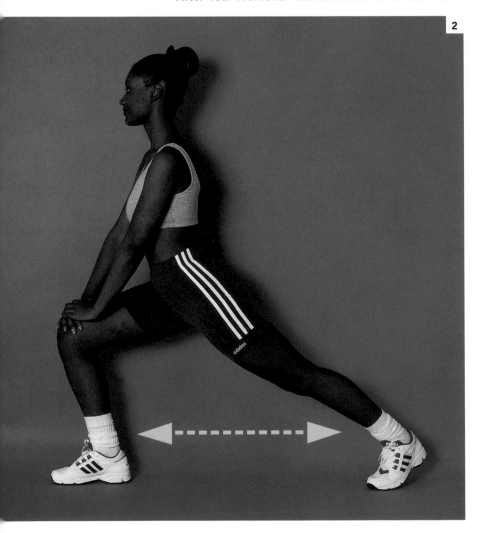

2

CHECKING YOUR FACTS

Because many of the stretches featured throughout this chapter are combination stretches, stretching out several muscles or body areas, the exact muscles stretched are not listed. If you need to know the muscle names, check the area of the stretch and refer to pages 10–11, where the annotated photographs will help you to identify the muscle groups used.

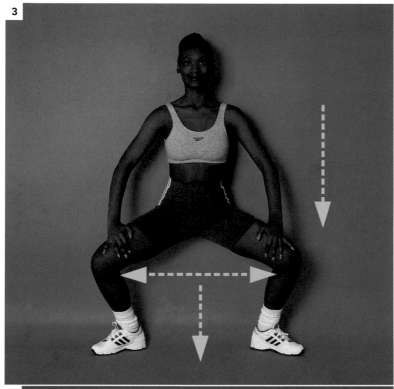

POSITION 3: **WIDE PLIÉ**

- Press the knees well out over the toes and make sure the feet are completely flat – no rolling!
- You should feel a stretch across the whole groin area.
- The lower you go in this position, the more you will increase the stretch.

Before Your Workout: Hold for 25 seconds.
After Your Workout: Hold for 30 seconds.

POSITION 4: **SPINE STRETCH**

- In this pose you are reaching up as high as you can, lifting the weight off the pelvis and ribcage and feeling the spaces between the vertebrae extend.
- Don't allow the back to arch too far, this is an upwards stretch.
- You should feel the spine lengthening, plus a stretch through the limbs – imagine that you are growing taller.

Before Your Workout: Hold for 25 seconds.
After Your Workout: Hold for 20 seconds.

Now that you have completed your basic stretch routine, move onto the mobilizers before you tackle your sports stretches.

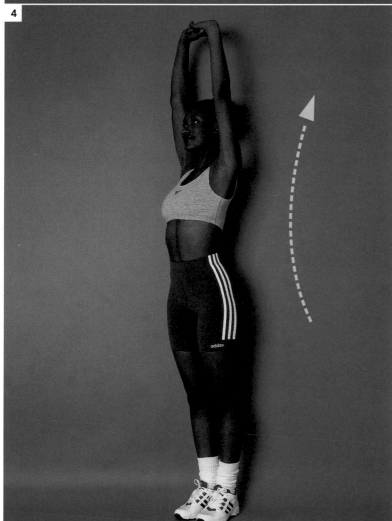

core **mobilizers**

POSITION 1:
KNEE CIRCLES

- Hold onto the knee caps and gently guide the knees in a clockwise direction and then back the other way. Bend the knees to help you.
- This will help warm up the knee and leg area.

Before Your Workout: Repeat 3–4 times in each direction.

DO THE TWIST

In order to get the most out of any twist move, one part of the body must be fixed so that the other part of the body has something to twist from or against. Usually, this means fixing the knees and hips in a forward-facing position and allowing the upper torso to rotate above it.

In this way the knee and hip joints are protected by not being pulled out of line.

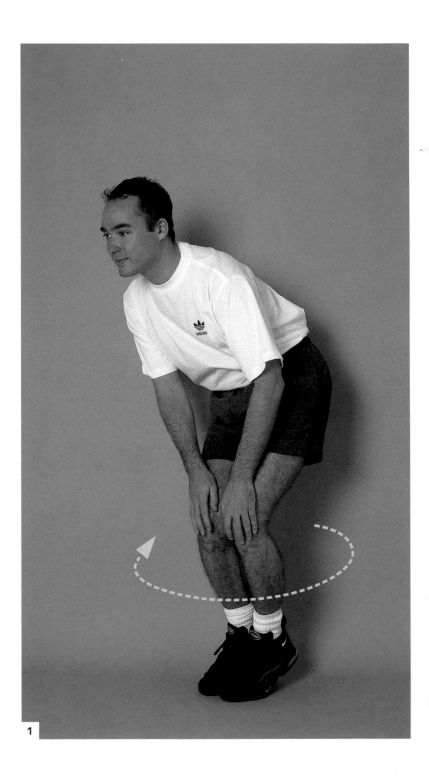

1

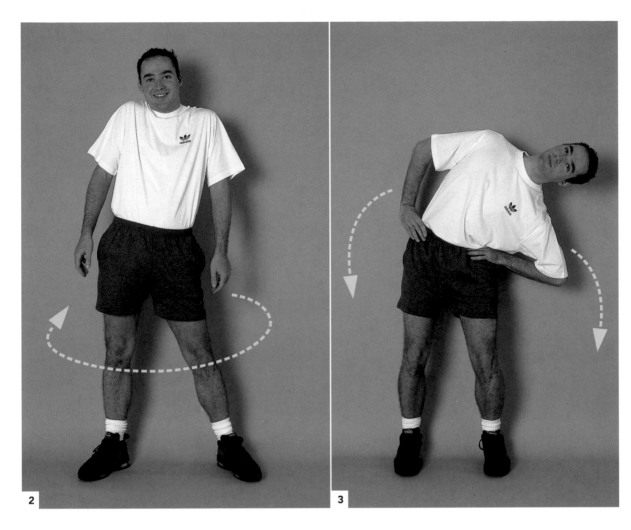

POSITION 2: **SHOULDER & HIP CIRCLES**

- Move the shoulders in large circles: hunch them right up to the ears, press them back behind you, squeezing the shoulder blades together, and then push them down and forwards. As you are doing this, circle your hips at the same time, moving them backwards out to one side and then around to the front and out to the other side.
- This will mobilize and loosen the shoulder and hip areas of the body.

Before Your Workout: Repeat 5–6 times in each direction. (Not needed as a cool-down.)

POSITION 3: **SIDE LEAN**

- Tip the top half of the torso from side to side, gently taking it slightly further each time.
- Do not flop; gently feel the stretch pulling up the sides of the torso.

Before Your Workout: Repeat 8–10 times.
After Your Workout: Repeat 4–5 times, more slowly.

Now that you have completed your basic stretch programme you can turn to your sports stretches to finish your pre- (and post-) stretch routine.

sports **stretches**

soccer stretches

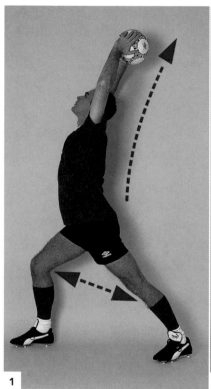

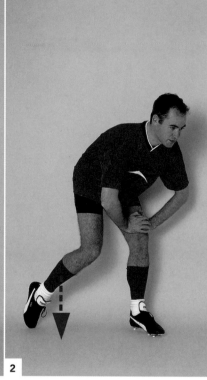

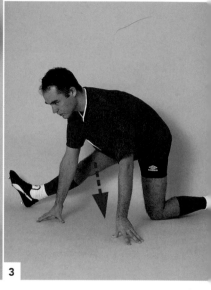

Look through all the sports, because you may find that a particular stretch in a sport you don't do is just as applicable to you in your chosen activity.

1

2

3

POSITION 1: **MOBILIZER**

Good for throw-ins and general flexibility on the field. Step into and out of this position.

Before Your Game: Hold for 30 seconds.

After Your Game: Hold for 35 seconds.

- Stretches the groin area and legs, chest and arms.

POSITION 2: **STRETCH**

Good for running and kicking moves.

Before Your Game: Hold for 25 seconds.

After Your Game: Hold for 30 seconds.

- Stretches the front of the lower leg and ankle.
- Keep the toes tucked underneath you as you press down on the back foot.

POSITION 3: **STRETCH**

Good for sliding tackles, high kicks and general flexibility on the field.

Before Your Game: Hold for 30 seconds.

After Your Game: Hold for 25 seconds.

- Stretches the groin area and back of thighs.

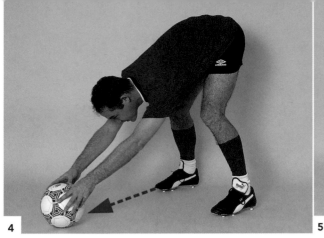

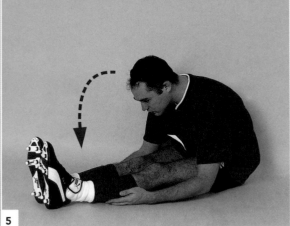

POSITION 4: **MOBILIZER**

Good for general flexibility to prevent injury, particularly to the hamstrings.

Before Your Game: Hold for 30 seconds.
After Your Game: Hold for 35 seconds.

- Stretches the lower back area and also along the backs of the legs.
- Try rolling the ball slightly away from you to increase the stretch in the lower back and then roll it in between the feet to feel more of a stretch at the back of the legs.

POSITION 5: **STRETCH**

Good for leg and back flexibility to prevent injury.

Before Your Game: Hold for 40 seconds.
After Your Game: Hold for 30 seconds.

- Stretches the backs of the legs and lower back. You may feel it in the calfs.

POSITION 6: **STRETCH**

Good for stretching out the buttocks for kicking and fast running.

Before Your Game: Using one hand for balance, hold for 30 seconds. Repeat on each leg.
After Your Game: Try adopting this same position sitting down on a warm surface and hold for 35 seconds. Repeat on each leg.

- Stretches the buttocks and side of thighs.

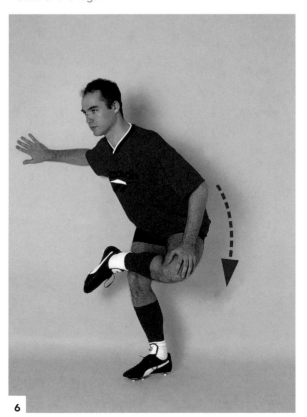

A LITTLE RELIEF

When you are performing the more extreme stretches, for any sport, a gentle rubbing or pummelling of the area stretched, after release, will help to bring blood to the area and provide instant relief for any discomforts.

american football
stretches

POSITION 1: **MOBILIZER**
Good for snaps and scrums

Before Your Game: Hold for 30 seconds each way.
After Your Game: Hold for 20 seconds.

• Stretches the chest, torso and hips.
• If you alternate from side to side quite quickly,
  this move will also serve as a mobility exercise,
  mobilizing waist and hips.

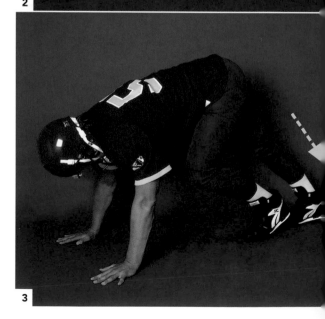

POSITION 2: **STRETCH**
This stretch is good for kicks, sprints and general
game flexibility.

Before Your Game: Hold for 30 seconds each leg.
After Your Game: Hold for 35 seconds each leg.

• Stretches the backs of legs and groin.
• You can put the ball in position to help you with the
  stretch or, if you want a greater stretch, then place
  the hands on the floor.

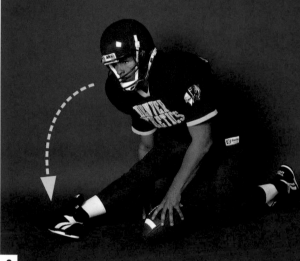

POSITION 3: **STRETCH**
Good for kicking, running and preventing injury to
the ankle area.

Gently press one heel into the floor while pressing
the ball of the foot into the floor and lifting the heel
of the other foot.

Before Your Game: Perform alternating presses for
1 minute.
After Your Game: Slow the movement down and
hold each foot down for 8 seconds each foot.
Repeat 5 times.

• Mobilizes ankles and stretches the Achilles tendons.

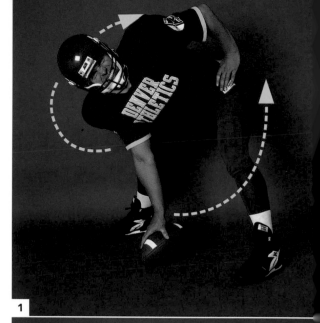

rugby
stretches

POSITION 1: **STRETCH**

Good for kicking, scrums and sprints.

Before Your Game: Hold for 40 seconds.
After Your Game: Hold for 35 seconds.

- Stretches the backs of the legs.
- Use the back of a chair or, if you're outdoors, use a tree or wall to let you bend forwards.

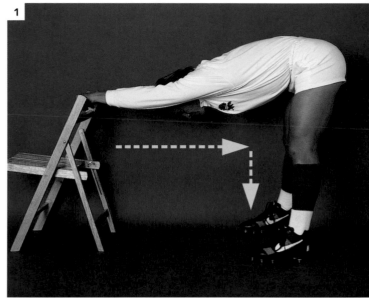

POSITION 2: **STRETCH**

Good for general game flexibility as well as for kicks and falls!

Before Your Game: Hold for 30 seconds each leg.
After Your Game: Hold for 35 seconds each leg.

- Stretches the buttocks and the side of the leg.
- The more you pull the legs towards you, the more you will feel a stretch.

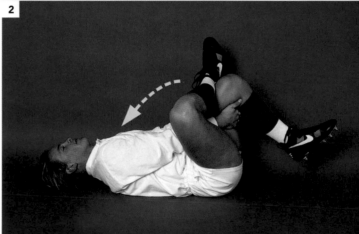

POSITION 3: **MOBILIZER**

Good for all the bending involved in scrums.

Swing the ball all the way up above the head and down between the legs, bending the knees.

Before Your Game: Swing the ball 15 times.
After Your Game: Swing the ball 10 times.

- Mobilizes the legs, hips and arms.

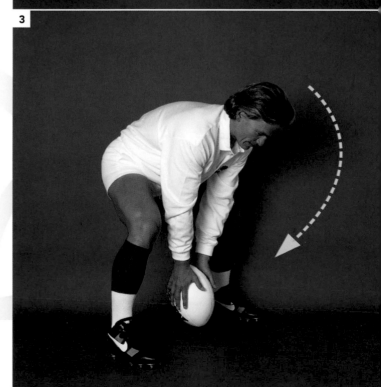

racquet
stretches

POSITION 1: **STRETCH**

Good for back-hand and net shots.

Before Your Game: Hold for 30 seconds each arm.
After Your Game: Hold for 35 seconds each arm.

• Stretches the shoulder and upper back.

POSITION 2: **STRETCH**

Good for serves and overhead smashes.

Before Your Game: Hold for 15–20 seconds.
After Your Game: Hold for 15 seconds.

• Stretches and limbers the back and spine.
• Ease the racket slowly down the back to increase the stretch. Keep the hips still and the pelvis tucked under.

POSITION 3: **MOBILIZER**

Good for alternating backhand and forehand shots.

Before Your Game: Swing and hold for 15 seconds each side, twice.
After Your Game: Hold for 20–30 seconds each side.

• Stretches the sides and front of the torso.

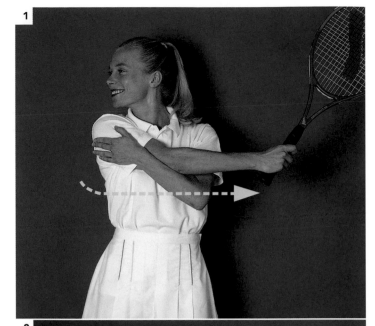

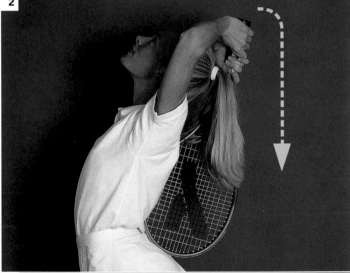

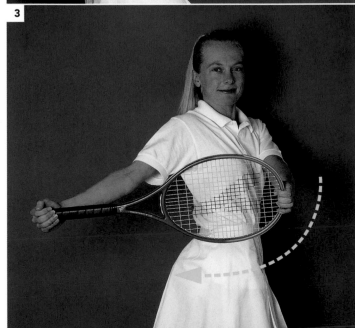

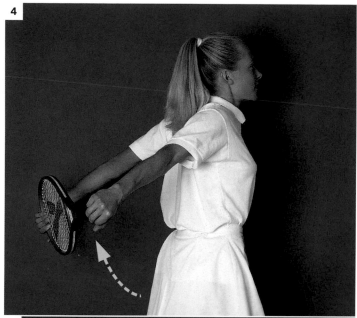

POSITION 4: **STRETCH**

Good for service swing and overhead shots.

Before Your Game: Hold for 20 seconds.
After Your Game: Hold for 20–30 seconds.

• Stretches the chest and arms and
  promotes shoulder mobility.

POSITION 5: **MOBILIZER**

Good for achieving a good grip, a strong
serve and general control of racquet.

Swing the racket over to one side, bringing it
horizontal, and hold; then swing back the
other way, bringing it again to a horizontal
position and holding.

Before Your Game: Repeat 8 times.
After Your Game: Repeat 8 times.

• Mobilizes the wrists and helps prevent
  strain in this area.

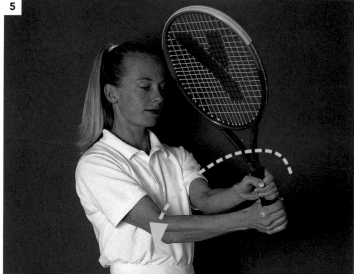

POSITION 6: **STRETCH**

Good for serve and overhead volley.

Bring the racquet forwards and then press it
back into the position shown, pressing as far
as your shoulders will allow.

Before Your Game: Repeat 10–12 times.
After Your Game: Hold for 15 seconds.
Repeat twice.

• Stretches and mobilizes the shoulders
  and promotes flexibility across the
  shoulder area.

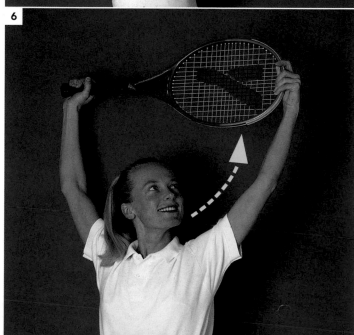

golf stretches

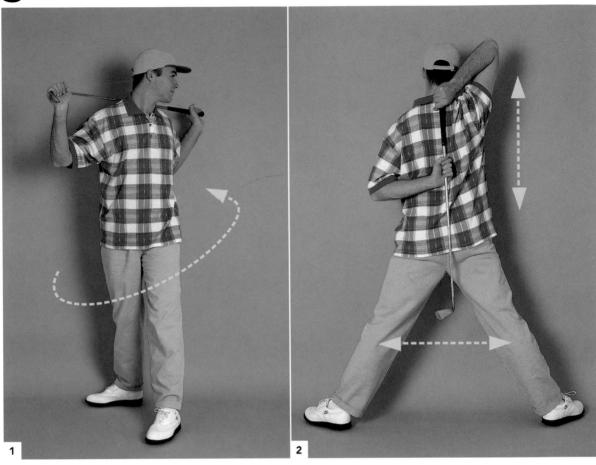

POSITION 1: **STRETCH**

Good for teeing off, as well as flexibility and ease of movement on all golf strokes.

Before Your Game: Twist one way and hold for 15 seconds.

After Your Game: Twist and hold for 20 seconds on each side.

• Stretches and mobilizes the torso and waist..
• Keep the hips facing forwards and make sure that the knees remain forwards and are not pulled out of line.

POSITION 2: **STRETCH**

Good for putting and pitching and driving from the tee.

Use your golf club to allow your lower arm to pull the top arm further back and so increase the stretch.

Before Your Game: Hold and pull down with the bottom hand for 10 seconds, then swap arm positions.

After Your Game: Hold for 15 seconds each arm.

• Stretches the shoulders and back of arm.
• Don't allow your back to arch as you reach behind.
• Keep your legs wide to provide an inner thigh stretch at the same time.

POSITION 3: **MOBILIZER**

Good for wrist flexibility, which is essential for control of putting and driving strokes.

Hold the club equally in both hands and lift and lower the wrists as far as possible each way, while keeping the forearms still.

Before Your Game: Flex up and down 15 times.
After Your Game: Flex up and down 20 times.

• Mobilizes and strengthens the wrists and forearms.

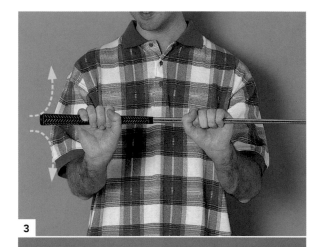

POSITION 4: **MOBILIZER**

Good for all-round playing flexibility.

Hold onto the club and give a real swing down and up to one side, letting the movement twist the body as it might in a real driving shot. Make sure, as you reach the top position (as in the photo), that you are fully stretched through your whole body and that there is a good twist in the waist.

Before Your Game: Swing to each side 8 times.
After Your Game: Swing to each side 8 times.

• Mobilizes the torso and legs.

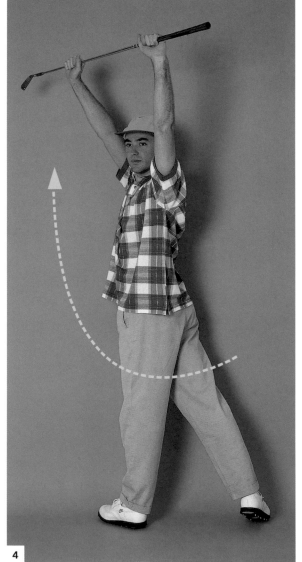

cricket and baseball stretches

All of these stretches apply to both sports

POSITION 1: **STRETCH**

Good for exactly what you might expect from the position – bowling – in both sports.

Start by going into the lunge position with back leg bent. Then reach the arm over towards your head to twist the torso slightly into a sideways leaning position.

Before Your Game: Hold for 20 seconds and repeat twice on each side.
After Your Game: Hold for 30 seconds on each side.

• Stretches the groin and the back, the Achilles and the side of the torso.

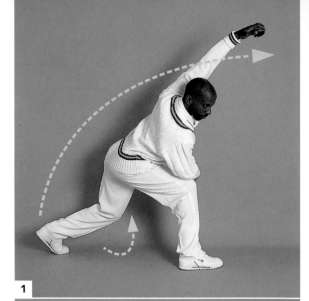

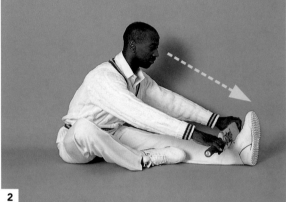

POSITION 2: **STRETCH**

Good for general leg flexibility for cricket and for runners' slide techniques in baseball.

Before Your Game: Hold for 30 seconds.
After Your Game: Hold for 40 seconds.

• Stretches the back of the straight leg and the outside thigh and buttock area of the bent leg.
• Use the bat to push yourself further down over the straight leg. When you have really developed your stretch, you can loop the bat over the foot to stretch even further!

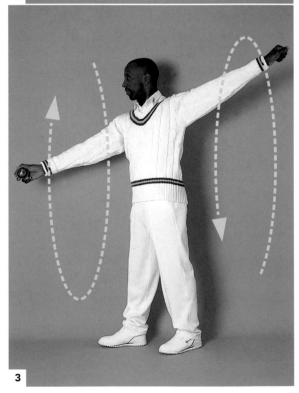

POSITION 3: **MOBILIZER**

Good for bowling, batting and throwing-arm mobility.

Start with both arms raised above the head and bring one forward as you press the other backwards so that each inscribes a full circle, passing each other at the top.

Before Your Game: Continue movement for 40 seconds.
After Your Game: Continue movement for 30 seconds.

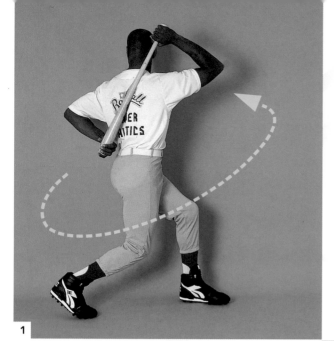

1

POSITION 1: **STRETCH**

Good for the wind-up bowl in baseball, batting in cricket and all the twisting movements involved in both sports.

Before Your Game: Twist and hold for 20 seconds on each side.
After Your Game: Twist and hold for 30 seconds on each side.

- Stretches shoulders and most of the upper torso; also mobilizes the legs and the hips.
- Pulling the bat up or down slightly while performing the stretch will increase the stretch on either shoulder.

POSITION 2: **STRETCH**

Good for twisting movements, for example the swing and follow-through for throwing, batting etc.

Before Your Game: Hold for 20 seconds on each side.
After Your Game: Hold for 40 seconds on each side.

- Stretches across the torso around to the lower back and also the buttock of the bent leg.
- If it is more convenient, do this position standing. Use the bat to pull that leg across the body, while keeping the opposite shoulder pressing back into the floor.

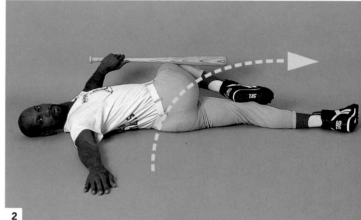

2

POSITION 3: **MOBILIZER**

Good for bending, scooping and running.

Bend into the squat position and then press the legs straight again, keeping your knees in line with your toes and without rolling on your feet.

Before Your Game: Perform 10 squats up and down.
After Your Game: Perform 3 squats slowly up and down.

- Mobilizes legs and hips and develops overall flexibility.
- Use the bat to provide counterbalance, so that you can really get the squat position correctly – that is, weight well over the heels as you bend the knees (not lower than 90 degrees).

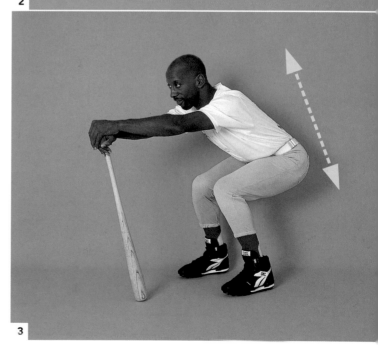

3

netball
stretches

POSITION 1: **STRETCH**
Good for catches and overhead throws.

Before Your Game: Hold for 15 seconds, repeat
5 times.
After Your Game: Hold for 20 seconds.

• Stretches the stomach and mobilizes the lower back.
• Use the weight of the ball to ease yourself gently
  backwards.

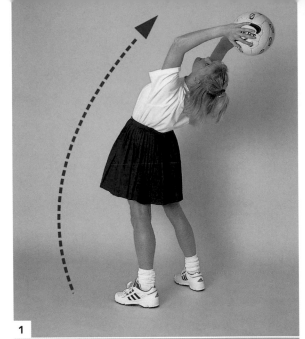

POSITION 2: **STRETCH**
Good for sprinting and jumping.

Before Your Game: Hold for 20 seconds on each leg.
After Your Game: Hold for 30 seconds each leg.

• Stretches the back of the thigh of the straight leg
  and the outside thigh of the bent leg. Also stretches
  across the upper back.
• Use the ball in this position to extend the stretch
  slightly further by rolling the ball away from you
  and then in again.

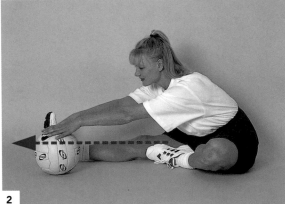

POSITION 3: **MOBILIZER**
This is an advanced mobilizer. Perform this carefully,
pulling up and in on the abdominals for support. Good
for throwing, kicking and fast bending movements.

Circle the ball all around the body in a complete circle.
Bend as much to the sides and back as you do to the
front.

Before Your Game: Circle one way 5 times and back
the other way 5 times.
After Your Game: Circle more slowly, 3 times each way.

• Mobilizes waist, hips and most of the torso.

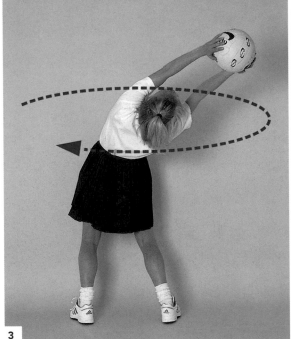

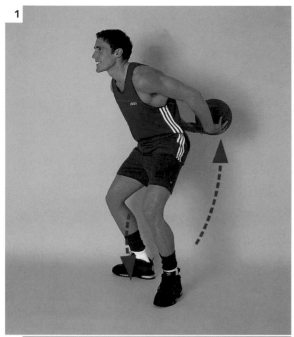

basketball
stretches

POSITION 1: **STRETCH**

Good for arm flexibility and throwing moves.

Before Your Game: Hold for 20 seconds and repeat twice.
After Your Game: Hold for 30 seconds and repeat twice.

- Stretches the chest and underarm/shoulder area and also warms the legs.
- Press the knees out over the toes as you lower into this plié position. Keep the hips in between the legs (as opposed to a squat, where the backside is behind the heels), then raise the ball as far behind you as you can, keeping the arms straight.

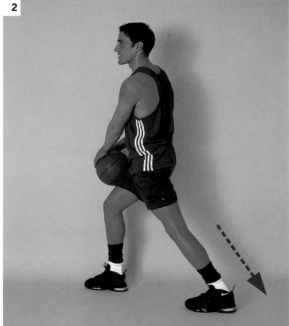

POSITION 2: **STRETCH**

Good for running, jumping and gaining speed.

Before Your Game: Hold for 20 seconds and repeat on each leg.
After Your Game: Hold for 30 seconds and repeat on each leg.

- Stretches the calf and Achilles tendon in the ankle (one of the few ligaments you can stretch slightly).
- This looks like a short lunge position, but the emphasis here is on the calf and ankle of the back leg. So bend your front knee and then press the back foot down slowly so that you feel a stretch in the calf muscles.

POSITION 3: **MOBILIZER**

Good for leaps, bends and dodges.

Start by holding the ball up high above the head, stretching through the spine. Now swing the ball down with arms outstretched and swing it between the legs, following with your head.

Before Your Game: Swing down and up 15 times.
After Your Game: Swing down and up 10 times.

- Mobilizes the hips, legs, arms and shoulders.

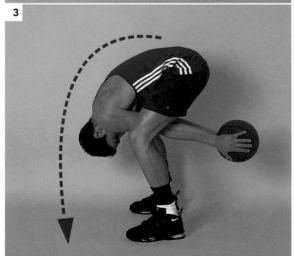

cycling
stretches

POSITION 1: **STRETCH**

This is an advanced stretch. Good for sustained cycling.

Before You Cycle: Hold for 10 seconds.
After You Cycle: Hold for 30 seconds.

- Stretches the front of the thigh.
- If you're outside, use a wall or tree to do this stretch against.

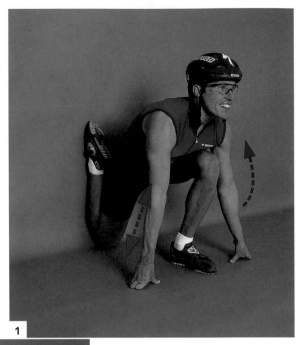

1

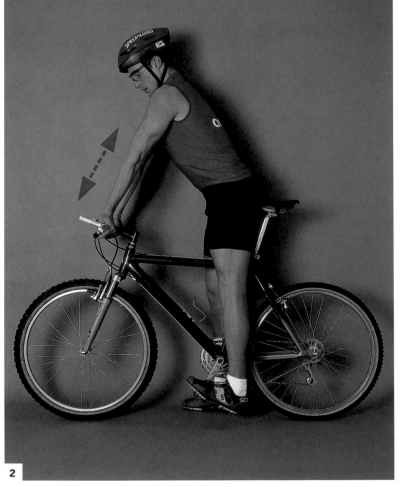

2

POSITION 2: **STRETCH**
Good for uphill riding and dismounts, and for when there is weight on the back wheel, which puts added stress on the back, Achilles area and calf.

Before You Cycle: Hold for 20 seconds on each leg and keep the arms in position to feel the stretch in the forearms.
After You Cycle: Hold for 30 seconds on each leg.

- Stretches the inside of the fore-arms and the Achilles and ankle.
- Note the position of the arms and the left leg and foot. This ensures that you are stretching two different areas at the same time.

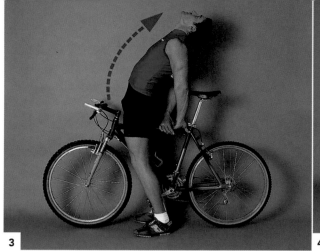

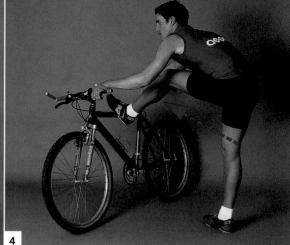

POSITION 3: **STRETCH**

Good for 'log hops', 'bunny hops' and wheel pivots, where the body is curved forward and the neck is pulling back on the shoulders. This stretch will help to redress the balance.

Before You Cycle: Hold for 10 seconds.
After You Cycle: Hold for 30 seconds.

- Stretches and limbers the lower back in opposition to the position that you must sustain constantly when actually cycling.
- You can hold onto the cross bar or the saddle, whichever is most comfortable in this position, but above all ensure that you are stable.

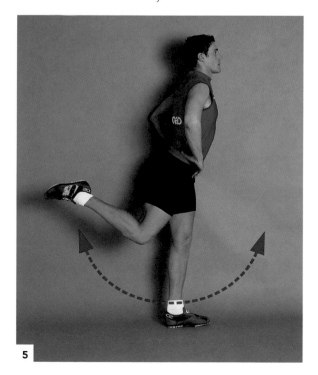

POSITION 4: **STRETCH**

Good for dismounting while moving and rising across a camber.

The first half of this exercise consists of lifting the leg up onto the cross bar with the leg bent, then for the second part, keep hold of the bike, and press it away from you by straightening the bent leg.

Before You Cycle: Hold the first position for 10 seconds, and then the second one for 15 seconds.
After You Cycle: Hold the first position for 15 seconds and then the second one for 25 seconds.

- Stretches the groin area at first and then, as you straighten, you will feel it at the back of the leg.

POSITION 5: **MOBILIZER**

Good for keeping the hips and legs mobilized.

Swing the leg forwards and back, keeping the hip from lifting and making sure that the movement is smooth.

Before You Cycle: Swing the leg gently each way 15 times.
After You Cycle: Swing the leg gently each way 25 times.

- Mobilizes the hips and gently stretches the back and front of the legs.

Note: *when riding downhill and doing rocks and drops, the shoulders are lower and the head is pulled back, so it is very important to stretch the neck. Pay particular attention to the neck stretch on page 110.*

swimming stretches

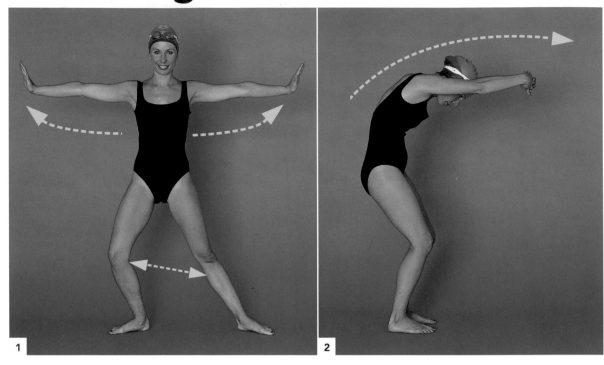

POSITION 1: **STRETCH**

Good for breast stroke and in-the-water flexibility.

Before Your Swim: Hold for 20 seconds.
After Your Swim: Hold for 30 seconds.

• Stretches the front of the upper arms and chest, also the groin and inner thigh area.

POSITION 2: **STRETCH**

Good for all of your strokes.

Before Your Swim: Hold for 20 seconds.
After Your Swim: Hold for 30 seconds.

• Stretches all across the upper back area.
• Hold your towel or clasp the hands to really make the most of this stretch.

POSITION 3: **STRETCH**

Good for freestyle stroke and general leg flexibility in the water.

Before Your Swim: Hold for 30 seconds each side.
After Your Swim: Hold for 40 seconds each side.

• Stretches the back of the straight leg, the outside of the bent leg and the torso.
• Make sure you get the twist on the upper body as well as the lean over towards the straight leg.

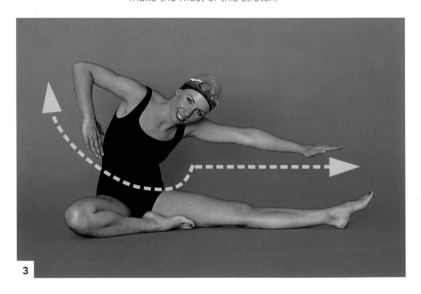

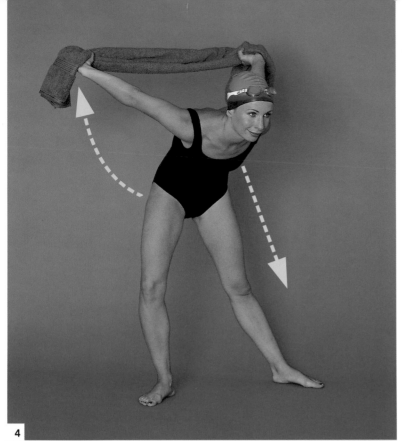

4

POSITION 4: **STRETCH**

Good for all strokes.

Make sure that you are in a stable lunge position. If you now tilt the hips slightly towards the bent leg, you will feel a stretch along the inner thigh of the straight leg.

Before Your Swim: Hold for 20 seconds. Repeat with lunge on the other side.
After Your Swim: Hold for 30 seconds. Repeat on the other side.

• Stretches the area underneath the shoulders as well as the inner thigh and groin area.
• Lift the arms as high as you can behind you to stretch out the shoulders and chest.

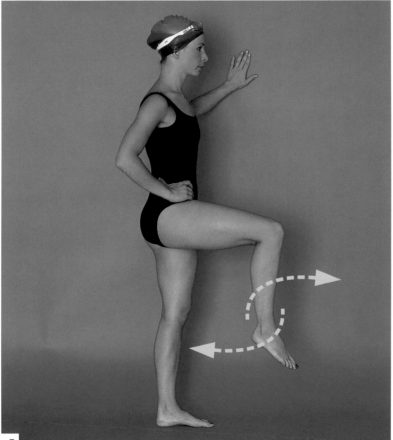

5

POSITION 5: **STRETCH**

Good for strong leg kicking and leg work in the water.

Standing in the water, simply flop your ankle backwards and forwards against the resistance.

Before Your Swim: Continue movement for 30 seconds on each leg.
After Your Swim: Continue movement for 40 seconds on each leg.

• The drag provided by the water will stretch the muscles around the ankle and gently massage the calf muscle.

skiing stretches

POSITION 1: **STRETCH**

Good for all the leg-work required in downhill skiing to keep you in a streamlined position. This stretch will exercise strong thighs and it will ensure that the large quadricep muscles are properly stretched out and so kept from becoming bulky or prone to cramp.

Before You Ski: Hold for 25 seconds on each leg.

For Your Après-ski: Hold for 35 seconds on each leg.

• Stretches the front of the thigh and the ankle of the bent leg.

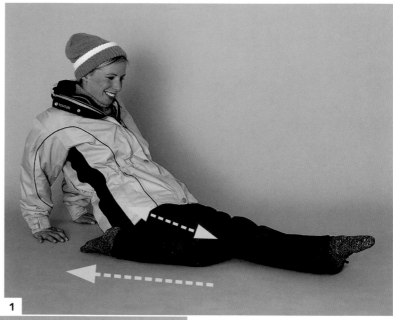

1

POSITION 2: **STRETCH**

Good for ankle mobility and general flexibility – ankles sustain quite a lot of pressure when skiing.

Before You Ski: Hold, with control, for 25 seconds.

For Your Après-ski: Hold for 35 seconds, resting your hands against a steady wall instead.

• Stretches the ankle and calves.

• You can do this stretch either in and out of skis, but you will get further with skis on because they support the forward incline. Make sure the rest of your body is taut and don't allow the stomach area to bow outwards.

2

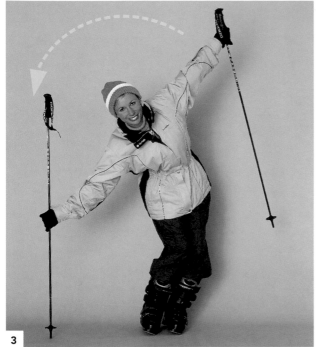

POSITION 3: **STRETCH**

Good for transversing moves and slide-slipping.

Before You Ski: Hold for 15 seconds.
For Your Après-ski: Hold for 35 seconds without boots on, keeping the ankles straight.

- Stretches the sides of the torso and the side of the leg and ankle.
- In ski boots you can do anything! As you take a curving bend over to one side, let your boots lean slightly to give you some stretch up the side of the ankle and use your pole, digging into the snow, to balance you. (If you do topple over, your hip should hit the snow first!)

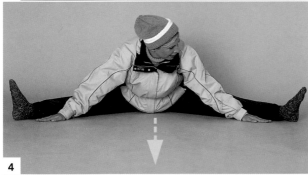

POSITION 4: **STRETCH**

Good for stretching out the inner thighs after all those static knee parallels and work with the quadriceps. Also good for snowploughing turns.

Before You Ski: Hold for 15 seconds.
For Your Après-ski: Hold for 35 seconds without boots on, keeping your feet pressed back as you lean forwards. Take this gently, as your inner thighs will be pretty tight after all that skiing.

- Stretches inner thighs.

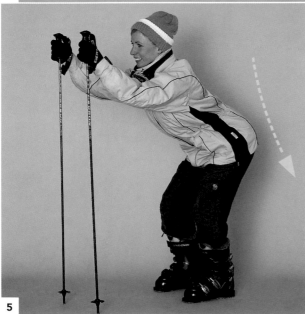

POSITION 5: **MOBILIZER**

Good for getting you used to the position for downhill slopes.

Before You Ski: Bend into this position and straighten again 8 times.
For Your Après-ski: Bend and straighten 6 times.

- Use the ski poles for balance, so that you can bend with the weight towards the heels. Keep the back straight and the abdominals pulled up.

dance and gymnastic stretches

POSITION 1: **STRETCH**

Good for all the basic moves in dance and gym.

Sit on both knees and then extend one leg straight back behind you, pressing that hip into the floor. Then bend the back leg up and pull the foot in toward your back.

Before Your Practice Session: Hold for 20 seconds each leg.
After Your Practice Session: Hold for 30 seconds each way then release and pummel the thighs.

• Stretches front of thighs and front of hips and gives a little flex to the lower back.

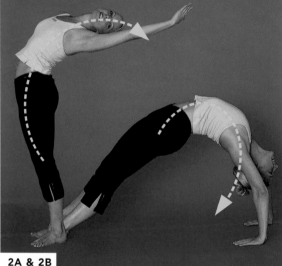

1

POSITION 2A AND 2B: **STRETCHES**

The first position here is more usual in dance, the second in gymnastics. Unless you are flexible, take great care.

Before Your Practice Session: Hold for 10 seconds and repeat 5 times.
After Your Practice Session: Hold for 20 seconds, and then roll the body into a ball, hugging the knees into the chest, and roll backwards and forwards to massage the lower back. Repeat 3 times.

• Stretches the abdomen and mobilizes the lower back.

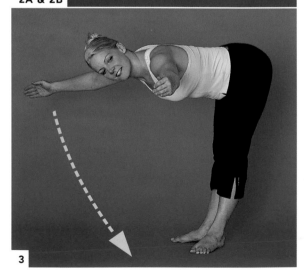

2A & 2B

POSITION 3: **MOBILIZER**

Good for getting your legs and back ready for action!

Start in an upright, perfect-posture position (Chapter 1). Reach the hands out to the side, or hold onto something with one hand, and lower the body slowly forwards. Keep your legs straight and the weight over the toes. Drop your head towards your knees and sweep your hand to the floor so that it just touches, then pull in on the abdominal muscles and curl the body back to the upright position.

Before Your Practice Session: Repeat the movement 3 times very slowly and with control.
After Your Practice Session: As above.

• Mobilizes and stretches the legs and lower back.

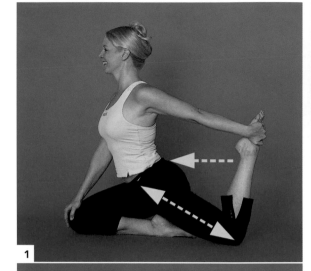

3

POSITION 4: **MOBILIZER**

Good for warming up the hips for fast, high kicks.

Move the bent knee in a figure 8, forwards and backwards. Keep the standing leg bent and hold onto something to keep your balance!

Before Your Practice Session:
Repeat the movement 8 times on each side.
After Your Practice: Repeat the movement 4 times, very slowly and with control.

• Mobilizes the hips.

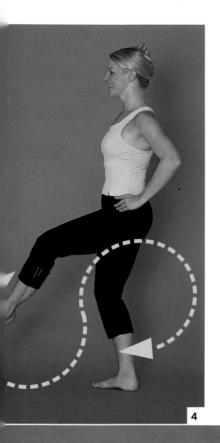

POSITION 5: **STRETCH**

Do this stretch only if you are feeling flexible. See page 107 for a description of how to get into the splits.

Good for making the legs flexible.

Start by adopting the lunge position, hands on the floor for support. Now gently slide your back leg away from you, taking your back foot as far away from the front one as it will go. Only go as low as is comfortable. If you go a little lower each time you will see improvement very quickly, and this is a good way to see just how flexible you are becoming.

Before Your Practice Session:
Hold for 10 seconds each leg.
After Your Practice: Hold for 30 seconds each way, then release and gently rub the groin area with your hands.

• Stretches the groin area, legs and inner thighs.

POSITION 6: **STRETCH**

Good for rapid movements and extreme stretch moves in gymnastics.

Start with legs as wide as possible and, with hands on the floor, slide the palms out as far as you can.

Before Your Practice Session:
Hold for 30 seconds.
After Your Practice: Hold for 30 seconds each way, then release and lightly pummel the groin and inner thighs with your fists.

• Stretches the groin area, legs and inner thighs.

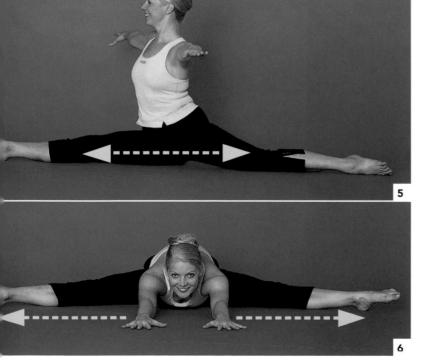

running
stretches

POSITION 1: **MOBILIZER**
Good for loosening the upper body muscles.

Move the elbow in a full circular motion first one way then the other. Make sure the elbow describes every part of the circle as you move it smoothly.

Before Your Run: Perform 8–10 times and repeat with other arm.
After Your Run: Perform more slowly 6–8 times.

• Mobilizes the arm and shoulder area.

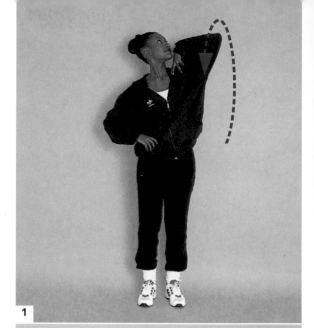

POSITION 2: **STRETCH**
Good for running, jumping and speed sports.

Seated in the position shown in the photo reach forwards as far as you can over your straight leg.

Before Your Run/Walk: Hold for 20 seconds and repeat on each leg.
After Your Run/Walk: Hold for 30 seconds and repeat on each leg.

• Stretches the hamstring and calf as well as the buttock and side of the bent thigh.

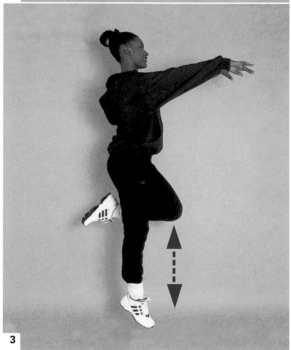

POSITION 3: **MOBILIZER**
Good for all running and walking actions of the legs.

Here you are simply swinging the arms as you push off the foot to effect a light jogging movement.

Before Your Run/Walk: Jog lightly 10–15 times.
After Your Run/Walk: Jog lightly 10–15 times.

• Mobilizes the legs, feet and ankles.

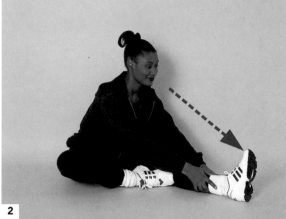

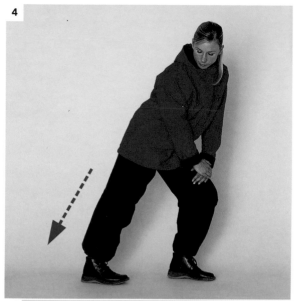

hiking
stretches

POSITION 4: **STRETCH**

Good for all running and walking actions of the legs.

Take a small lunge position here, but put the emphasis on feeling the stretch in the back of the calf on the back leg.

Before Your Run/Walk: Hold for 20–30 seconds and repeat on each leg.
After Your Run/Walk: Hold for 20–30 seconds and repeat on each leg.

• Stretches the calf and Achilles tendon (which will stretch slightly).

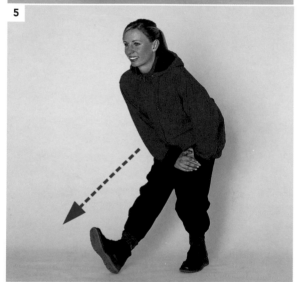

POSITION 5: **STRETCH**

Good for all running and walking actions of the legs and helps prevent cramp and injury to the back of the legs.

Adopt the position as shown in the photo with hands resting on the bent knee for support. Press forward to feel the stretch up the back of the leg.

Before Your Run/Walk: Hold for 20–30 seconds.
After Your Run/Walk: Hold for 20–30 seconds and repeat on each leg.

• Stretches the hamstrings.

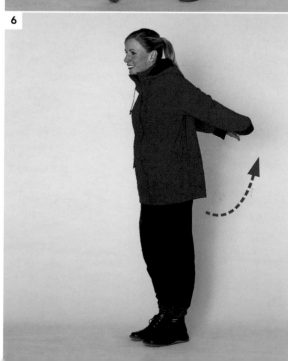

POSITION 6: **MOBILIZER**

Mobilizes arms for sudden or reaching actions.

Lift the arms behind you as high as you can to mobilize the shoulder joints.

Before Your Run/Walk: Lift as high as you can, and lower with a brief hold 15 times.
After Your Run/Walk: Lift and hold for longer, even tipping your arms right over your head (and bending the knees) to really increase the stretch (see page 42).

• Mobilizes the shoulders and arm area.

ballistic
stretch

Ballistic stretching means "bouncing" from an initial stretch position in order to increase the stretch further. Some sports use ballistic-style movements as a substantial part of their repertoire. The kicks, head and back-flicks made by dancers, the jumps and whips of the gymnast and the explosive punch-kicks of the martial artist, all call upon lightning speed extension of the muscles. In these sports then, it is essential to put your body through some of these fast movements in the warm-up phase to prevent injury.

SOME BAD REVIEWS

In recent years, the ballistic stretching method has received a lot of bad press in the fitness world. Although it is popular in certain disciplines, there are various problems associated with this approach, as many physiotherapists have pointed out:

- Any rapid stretch without warning will activate the stretch reflex (see page 22) and make the muscle tense up rather than encouraging it to release.
- Rapid bouncing, using your body weight, may take the movement out of your control, so that it is difficult to stop the movement before any damage occurs. What happens then is that small tears (micro traumas) occur that can lead to a build-up of scar tissue. This, in turn, may ultimately lead to less flexible muscles – the exact opposite of what you are aiming to achieve!

ON THE PLUS SIDE

On the "pro" side, some physiotherapists suggest that:

- If you do ballistic movements in a gentle, controlled way, you can retrain the stretch reflex so that it doesn't occur while you are doing the movement.

- Some of the ballistic-style movements also provide the body with speed and mobility. For example, leg swings allow the legs to stretch and mobilize at the same time.

"ROCK" NOT "SHOCK"

Ballistic stretching – a certain amount of moving within a position in order to push the stretch a little further or so you can become comfortable with the stretch you are in – can have lots of benefits.

Take, for example, a stretch for the inner thighs where you are sitting with your legs straight and out to the side, and you wish to reach further over one leg and then into the middle. Rather than going straight into the full stretch over one leg, it is far better to start by rocking the body from side to side. This is similar to a certain mobilizing exercise, where the body is given a warning in the areas about to be used and there is some build-up of heat in the hip joints. Similarly, when starting to stretch forwards, if you put your hands on the floor in front of you and rock gently backwards and forwards, these little pressing movements will warm up the inner thighs before you push as far forwards as you can go.

TAKING IT FURTHER

With this type of stretching, once you stretch to your initial limit, you can then do some more gentle rocking to help you become used to that position – and eventually you may go a bit further. The thing to remember when rocking or doing little pushes is that your hands should always be on the floor to support you as a safeguard against going too far. In this way you are always in control. Used carefully and correctly, these gentle rocking movements can really help your body acclimatize to the stretch and distract your mind so that the stretch can be maintained. (See Chapters 2 and 3 for more information on exactly how to stretch.)

At all times do try to remember that stretching is a gradual process and that no amount of forcing, bouncing or bending will stretch the muscles in one session. In fact if you push things too far you are prone to over stretching and thus "pulling" or even tearing a muscle. Always work slowly and conscientiously toward your goals, making the process a regular event rather than a forced one-off session.

CHECK IT OUT

If you find that you are very stiff or that over the course of weeks your stretch ability is not improving, it may be worth a trip to the physiotherapist just to check there are no anatomical restrictions or other conditions that may be limiting your progress. Young, as well as older people can suffer from various forms of arthritis, which tend to cause undue stiffness in the joints, and if this were to be the case then your physio might even recommend some gentle stretches to help the condition. Most people, however, need nothing more than a regular stretch programme worked into their lives.

THE BEST PROGRAMME

Throughout this book there have been many different methods of stretching detailed. It is up to you to try as many ways as you can and find the ones which work best for you. People who have come from competitive sports background, particularly those in martial arts, gymnastics and dance will be accustomed to stretching in a somewhat ballistic mode and this may be the method that appeals to them most. Their bodies will be used to the feelings of stretch and they will have learned how far they can go with extending the stretch.

Others who are less familiar with the whole concept of stretching may find any kind of stretch very painful at first. This is because the body is feeling something unfamiliar and it will take time for the body and mind to relax with the sensations and learn not to panic. That is why a gradual build-up is such a good idea. It is also a good idea to use the different methods of stretch at different times. If you are feeling full of energy and raring to go one morning, you may want to make your session more dynamic by adopting stretch positions and moving around in them to become really at ease. You may also be in the mood to try the moving sequences in Chapter 6 which give you the opportunity to make your stretch programme a fun and creative experience! These kinds of stretches are also good to do with children. On the other hand if you are just starting to move in this way again, after a long break or an injury then the levelled programmes will help you progress along with the relaxation stretches in Chapter 6. Relaxing in a stretch position will allow your body to learn that stretch need not be painful or awkward, but can help relieve stiffness in a non-threatening way.

If you have worked hard for a week or so and your body is feeling a little jaded, use some of the partner stretches to re-enthuse yourself and make the session really fun! Then get your partner to try out some of the massage techniques mentioned to entirely relax those muscles!

5 CHAPTER stretching with a partner

This chapter is all about stretching with a friend. There are many ways that two people can work together to bring variety to their stretch routines and increase their stretching potential as they do so. Working with a partner can help you stay motivated longer and have fun at the same time!

Sometimes it can be difficult to get your body into certain stretch positions. A partner can help in this process, acting rather as a personal instructor would, by checking the body position, guiding a limb to its correct placement, and ensuring that there are no jerky movements and so less risk of injury. They can also provide some massage and a post-stretch rub down – which always feels better when it is done by someone else!

DOS AND DON'TS

When you are stretching with a partner, there are some important points that you must bear in mind for your safety.

Communication is vital when you are working with someone else's body. Remember, you cannot feel what your partner is feeling – only by talking to them and listening to exactly what they say will you be able to maintain the right degree of control. Whenever you begin to help your partner to stretch out, keep your mind on what you are doing and constantly ask them how they are feeling.

If you are the 'presser', as opposed to the person being stretched, check your partner's posture before you begin and during the stretch; make sure that there is no slouching or tendency to favour one side of the body. Once in a stretch position, the person being stretched is often less aware of his or her position than you will be.

The presser must also check their partner's breathing. Breathing during

partner stretching should be normal and regular, with no held breaths. Occasionally, you may direct them to inhale strongly and exhale slowly, to aid the stretch. The instructions on the following pages will indicate when this is appropriate.

BODY TALK

As you practice your partner stretching techniques, you will find that you become more adept at listening, and even feeling, your partner's body signals. When you first press your partner into a position, for example, you will feel the resistance in that person's muscles. As you continue to hold, and the stretch reflex becomes de-activated, you will feel a slight "give" in the muscles. To begin with, you will have to ask your partner exactly what she or he is feeling, but after a while you will start to recognize the signs – just as you learn to feel what is comfortable for your own body you will know when a muscle is releasing, when it is tiring and so on.

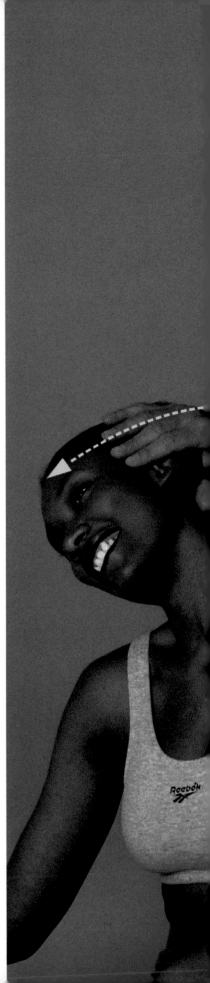

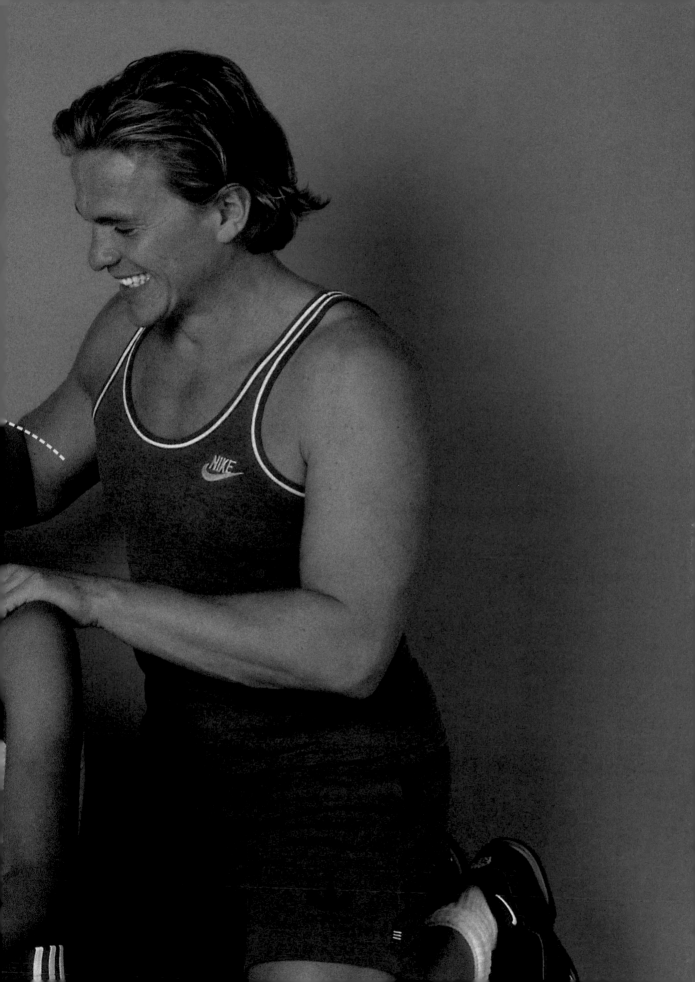

Remember also to check that your partner's breathing is slow and rhythmical. They should not be holding their breath – if they are then they are obviously tense and not relaxed in the position. Also, always keep talking to your partner throughout and make sure that they are talking back.

PARTNER STRETCHING TECHNIQUES

When starting to stretch a partner, you must understand that quite a large amount of pressure is normally needed. Most bodies are heavy – and limbs are surprisingly heavy! So when manipulating another person into a position, it is important to handle them firmly and with confidence. It is always better if the two people stretching each other are relatively similar in height and weight. If you are not, don't worry, but make sure that the heavier person takes extra care.

THE ART OF TOUCH

Don't be afraid to touch and grasp your partner, and don't shrink from pressing firmly when the following pages indicate that is necessary. Usually, the positions where you can

---

A HELPING HAND

Gentle manipulation of a certain area by someone else will often help to relieve any superficial stiffness, discomfort or injury, and it may be that a partner can work on areas that are too difficult for you to reach properly yourself (see Chapter 6). Any major injuries, such as breaks or sprains – or areas that you think may be badly injured – must, of course, be looked at by a qualified medic. Do not try to act as each other's physiotherapist.

---

do this best are those where you have the ability to use your own body weight to increase your partner's stretch range.

STAYING WITH IT

With partner stretches, the stretch needs to be maintained for some time, usually 20–50 seconds, so that the developmental phase of the stretch can be activated. This is when you feel (or your partner will tell you) that the muscle has started to release slightly. At this point, you can take the stretch a little further, allowing your weight to go over a little more as you feel your partner's muscles letting you do so. Always make sure, however, that you are in control of your own weight, and therefore have the ability to pull away from your partner if necessary.

LETTING GO

If your partner expresses discomfort at any time, or at the end of the stretch, the way you release your partner is as important as the way you apply the pressure. Never just jump away from the stretch you have made, but withdraw gently and firmly, so that the muscle stretch releases gently too. Jumping back from pressing – for example if your partner suddenly says "ow!" – is much more likely to distress the muscle because it springs back too quickly. Always release the hold slowly. Withdraw the pressure in a slow, controlled manner, or ask your partner to press against you to start the withdrawal. In this way, your partner's muscles will have time to readjust and "understand" that the pressure has been released. Your partner may then need to take a few seconds to relax and recover. You can aid him by gently rubbing

the muscles you have stretched, bringing blood and warmth to the area. Keep chatting to your partner and check that his muscles feel back to normal before embarking on the next stretch. Or swap around so that he can repeat the stretch for you before you start on him again! This gives time for each muscle group being stretched to recover.

One of the most exciting ways to stretch is to use the PNF method outlined opposite – which really is easier when you have a partner. Some of the stretches featured over the following pages use this method, and you will see how it really extends the limits of your stretching capabilities.

PNF
stretching

Proprioceptive Neuro-muscular Facilitation (PNF) was adapted from physiotherapy techniques that were developed to help stroke patients. PNF works on two basic principles:

1. If a muscle is contracted hard for at least 10–20 seconds, then immediately afterwards the tone of the muscle will decrease briefly. If a stretch is applied at this point, it will allow a greater range of motion.

2. When a muscle is contracted, the opposing muscle releases and the tone of that muscle decreases, briefly allowing greater stretch – known as reciprocal inhibition.

There are two ways to carry out PNF stretches:

1. By using the muscle in a vigorous isometric (held) position for some time

2. By using the opposing muscle group in the same way.

When you release the hold, the sustained tension will facilitate a greater stretch. Remember when using this method that you should warm up thoroughly first. Warm muscles can contract much more, and for longer – which is necessary for this way of working – and they will stretch further afterwards.

PUSHING FURTHER

You will find that a partner is especially helpful for the second method, giving you someone to push against initially. And when you release the pressure, you have your partner to guide your limbs through the greater range of motion that you have just gained.

This method is particularly good for areas where stiffness is a stubborn problem. When you feel you really cannot go any further in a stretch in a particular set of muscles (the hamstrings, for example, are particularly inflexible), PNF stretching can help you find new stretch in those muscles – if done regularly and responsibly. This type of stretching will also add variety to your stretch workout, as it concentrates the mind and works the opposing muscles, so you will be toning some of your muscles at the same time.

Turn to the following pages to try a variety of partner stretches that are fun, safe and bound to extend you!

It is possible to attempt PNF stretching on your own, although it is much easier, and probably safer, to do it with a partner to guide you. If you are on your own, try a few different ways of feeling the syndrome just to get you used to the idea. See 'A Case in Point' box. Also try the following.

Sit in a comfortable position, with one leg outstretched and resting on a couple of cushions or a low step. This allows the leg to be raised slightly off the floor so that you can press down with some force. Now press the foot down towards the floor as if you were trying to push it through the cushions! Maintain this tension for 30–50 seconds, but be careful not to push through the back of the knee too much. You should not feel the back of the knee being stressed, so try to keep the tension in the quadriceps (front of thigh muscles). Now release the tensions and, taking hold of the working leg, roll onto your back and pull the straight leg in towards your nose as far as it will go. Hold momentarily and then release. Roll back to an upright sitting position to repeat the process again. If you repeat this three times, you should notice a distinct increase in how far your leg can be pulled towards your nose from the time you started to the time you finished. Repeat the whole process regularly for lasting benefit.

A CASE IN POINT

As a child, did you ever play the game where you stand in a doorway and push your arms against the door frame as hard as you can for a minute? Try it now. When you walk away from the door, your hands will float upwards as if they are weightless and have a mind of their own. ("Magic!" We used to exclaim as children.) This is reciprocal inhibition in action.

1. THE BRIDGE

Have your partner sit comfortably, with the soles of his feet touching each other and legs bent, with knees falling out to the side. The feet don't need to be pulled in tightly towards the groin but should be placed quite far out in front, so that he is relaxed. Your partner should sit with a straight back, lifting up through the spine from the hips, and take a deep breath in and then one out.

Position yourself directly behind your partner, sitting high up on your knees, so that, when force is required, you are in a position to apply it. Now, the person being stretched should place his hands on his ankles – not around his feet – and relax his back so that he curls slightly forwards. With your right

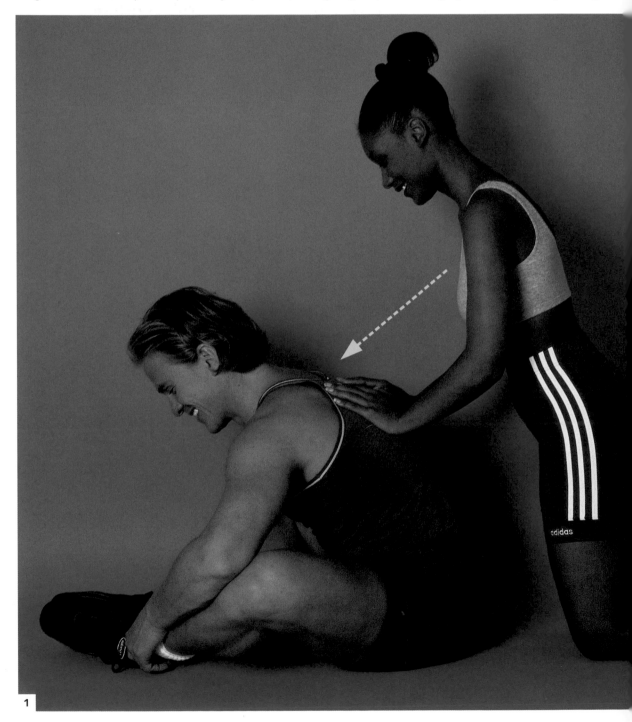

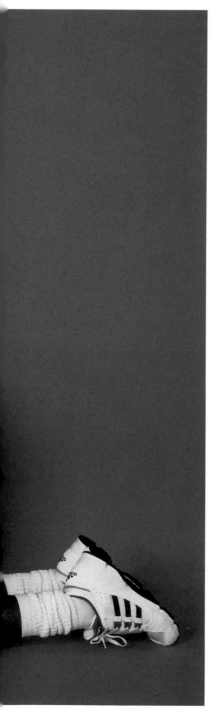

hand, press firmly on his lower back and, with the flat of your hand, try to press your partner further forwards from the base of his spine. You will probably find that your partner does not move all that far as you do this. Although this spot is where stretches should begin from, most people in fact need the pressure further up the spine in order to help them bend forwards.

Next, take your left hand and press the middle of your partner's back to apply pressure gently but firmly, easing them a little further forwards. Finally, still maintaining the pressure, place both hands wherever the back is highest – it should still be curved – and press firmly with both hands until your partner tells you he has reached his conformable limit.

Once you have reached this position, hold for 20–30 seconds. Now ask your partner to press his back against your palms as if to push you upwards. Resist the push for several seconds and then gently allow your partner to press himself to sitting and recover. After this stretch, let your partner bring his knees together and, sitting with his hands behind for support, have him tip his knees from one side to the other to help him recover from the sustained pressure.

THE PRESSER

While you are exerting pressure on your partner, be very aware of how he might be feeling. Talk to him, particularly as you push him over, and ask if he is comfortable. If you feel, during the 30-second hold, that your partner's muscles have relaxed, then go with this and take your pressure lower as his muscles allow you to. Once you have gone lower, however, don't allow your partner to lift up again. Hold it there. Never force your partner lower than you feel his muscles will allow.

At the end of some of the following stretches, you may need to help your partner come back to the original position. Or try asking him to push against you, which will signal to his muscles that the stretch has ended. Take a few moments to allow your partner to recover and move around to release tension.

THE STRETCHEE

It is very important to try and relax your muscles and to have faith in your partner to stretch you out responsibly and with delicate care. If you don't have complete trust in your partner, you will not be able to relax fully – unless you do, you will not get the greatest possible benefit from such a programme.

Take slow, deep breaths and concentrate on telling your muscles not to fight the pressure but instead to r-e-l-e-a-s-e.

As well as talking to your partner and keeping her informed of what you are feeling, you also need to have your own internal dialogue going to encourage and reassure your own body! In this way your brain will learn to let your muscles release without fear of injury.

SAFETY FIRST

If, at any time, you feel your partner is pushing you too far, try using these code words:

- "HOLD", telling your partner to maintain the stretch.
- "ENOUGH", telling your partner to withdraw pressure slowly and gently.

Above all, don't panic when you feel the stretch reflex activate and the muscles initially tighten and pull away. Keep the communication going with your partner, and with yourself, breathe deeply, and remind and reassure yourself that you will soon become accustomed to the sensation.

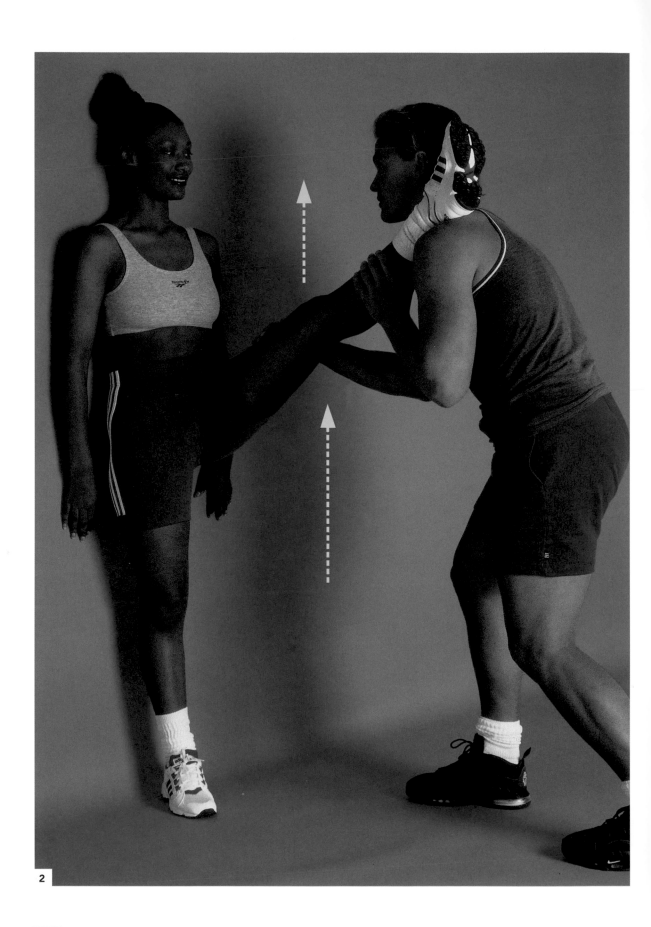

2

2. THE MAGIC LAMP

This stretch uses the second PNF method of stretching described earlier in this chapter (page 85).

METHOD

Basically, the principle here is to use your partner's resistance to allow you to push hard with the top of your thigh so that your quadriceps are in a strong contraction for some seconds. When you release the back of the leg, the hamstring muscle will be that much more supple. If you repeat this stretch pattern up to three times on each leg, you will really notice the difference in the stretch you have obtained; from the time you start to the time you complete the last movement.

THE STRETCHEE

The person being stretched stands with her back to a wall and presses her heels and bottom in tight to that wall. Place the hands either side to aid balance. Now bend your leg and lift your foot off the floor to "give" one leg to your partner. Allow your partner to lift that leg as high as it will go naturally. You should not feel that he is forcing it at this stage, you should simply feel that he has lifted it to its natural limit. Make sure that your other foot is flat on the ground, your bottom is not being pulled away from the wall, and your stomach is not sagging.

Now take a deep breath in and, as you exhale, start to exert force with your lifted leg, trying to force it down towards the ground. Use the muscles on the top of the thigh – look at these muscles, concentrate on them and press hard for 50 seconds. If you are pressing hard enough, your partner should have a hard time keeping that leg up there!

Make sure you don't feel too much of a push through the joint of the knee. Try to keep the pressing leg just slightly bent and concentrate on using the quadriceps to exert force. Keep breathing at all times while your partner counts out 50 seconds. When he tells you to release, stop pushing immediately and just allow your limb to be lifted.

THE PRESSER

The presser starts by holding his partner's leg in both hands and lifting it as far as it will naturally go. Bend your knees and pull in on the stomach to give yourself support – once there is pressure on that leg you will find it really hard work!

Now time 50 seconds on your stopwatch and hold your partner's leg where it is, as she pushes downwards. Don't try to lift the leg any higher – simply resist her attempts to push it down to the floor. Keep both arms bent as you resist the push, so that you are taking the weight in your arms and not in the spine. After 50 seconds, ask her to release. As you feel the pushing cease, wait 5 seconds and then gently lift the leg between 2 and 3 inches higher.

You should now find that the leg will lift a few extra inches quite effortlessly. Don't push it any further than this but simply take the leg to its new natural height and ask your partner to start pushing again. Repeat the process two more times, followed by a gentle lift each time to extend the muscle. Repeat on the other leg and then swap roles.

By the end of the stretch, your leg will probably have gone from, say, a 90-degree angle to one of 110 degrees. This is where the use of the quadriceps has allowed a greater

stretch to take place in the opposing muscles – in this case the hamstrings. Because many people experience stiff legs, this is a really good stretch to help extend your flexibility. It is particularly useful to be working with a partner because lifting your own leg into a position it doesn't want to reach is pretty difficult.

Remember, to capitalize on the increased flexibility you have gained, you must repeat this process often. In this way the legs get used to stretching and the flexibility will last.

As you feel your flexibility increasing with this method, you can go on to try other stretches with your legs. Try the splits practice on page 107, as you should now find this exercise easier and may get lower than when you first attempted it. In addition, remember that the Magic Lamp stretch can also be used to lift the legs to the side, so that you are stretching the adductor muscles as well. Perform the same sequence as in the main example, but stand with the side of your body pressed to the wall and have your partner lift the leg in a forward diagonal. The leg should lift to the side, without hitching the hip up.

You could also try a similar PNF stretch where you are seated with your legs open and touching your partner's (see photograph on page 91). In this position, you would squeeze in with both your legs and then release and allow your partner to ease your legs outwards.

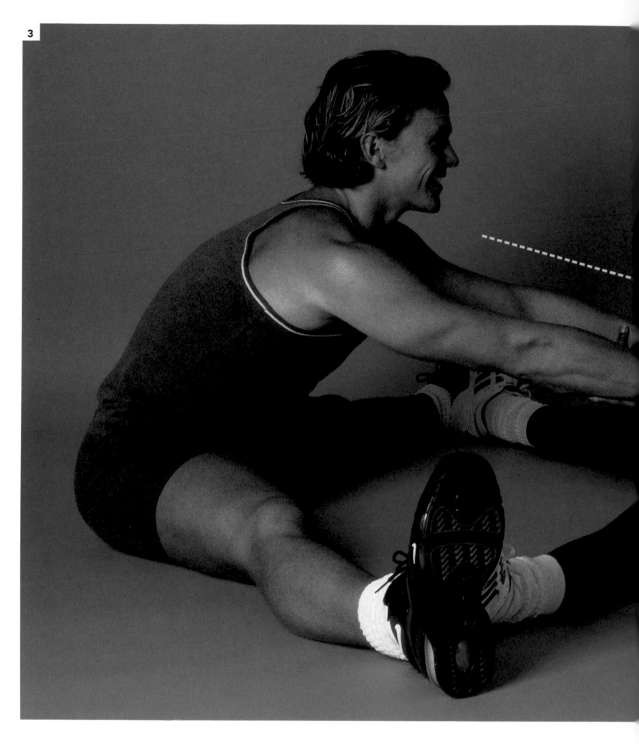

3. THE ROWBOAT

This stretch routine allows both partners to stretch out the other person's inner thigh muscles with enough force to make a real difference in the stretch, but with as little risk of injury as possible.

STARTING POSITION

Both partners sit on the floor facing one another and with their feet out as far to each side as is naturally comfortable. The presser places her feet against her partner's ankles and keeps her knees bent. Then the presser supports herself with her hands behind her and straightens her legs by pushing the legs of her partner further outwards in a smooth movement. Now the stretchee and presser join hands while grasping each other's wrists securely.

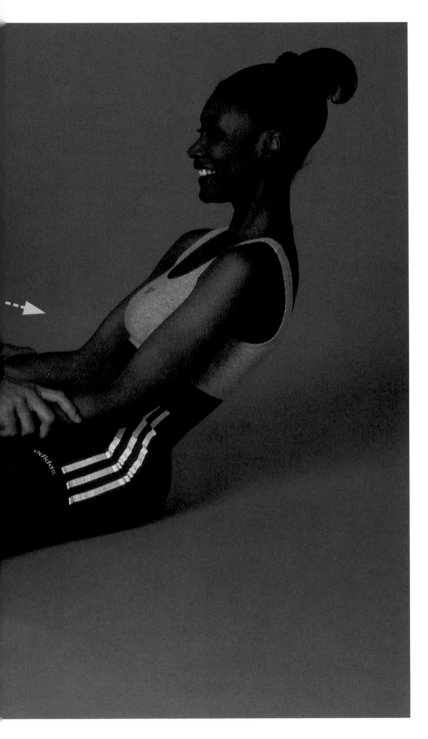

his legs stable with your feet. Hold this lean for 15–20 seconds and then lean forwards and allow your partner to lean back himself, feeling the stretch in your own thighs. Hold for just a few seconds and then lean backwards once more on your side.

THE STRETCHEE

As your partner leans back, allow yourself to be pulled forwards and feel the stretch in your inner thighs. Keep your back as straight as possible and keep the stomach lifted so that there is no pulling on your lower or upper back. If you feel you are being pulled too far, use the code words "hold" or "enough" to give yourself a breather before you try again. As you hold the stretch position, breathe normally and try to relax the legs as they are stretched. When your partner eases forwards, use this as your cue to pull gently with your arms and then start to lean backwards – not too far – to give your partner a gentle stretch.

With one partner as the stretchee, rock gently backwards and forwards 3 times before resting and swapping roles. When you wish to change roles, remember to change the foot position so that one person is being stretched further than the other. Try to do this stretch together as part of your regular stretch programme. (If you don't always have a partner, you can try doing the same sort of stretch by pushing your feet against the wall and leaning towards it.)

After the stretch, bring your legs together. Now, gently massage both of your inner thighs with the palms of your hands, or lightly pummel the muscles there to bring the blood to these areas and, in doing so, relieve any held-in tension there may be.

THE PRESSER

Now, holding onto your partner's arms securely and, keeping your stomach well lifted and your back straight, start to lean slowly backwards, pulling your partner easily and gently towards you. Use the strength of your arm to ease your partner towards you.

Keep talking to your partner the whole time, so that you know how much of a stretch he is feeling. As you lean backwards, you stretch your partner's inner thighs, while keeping

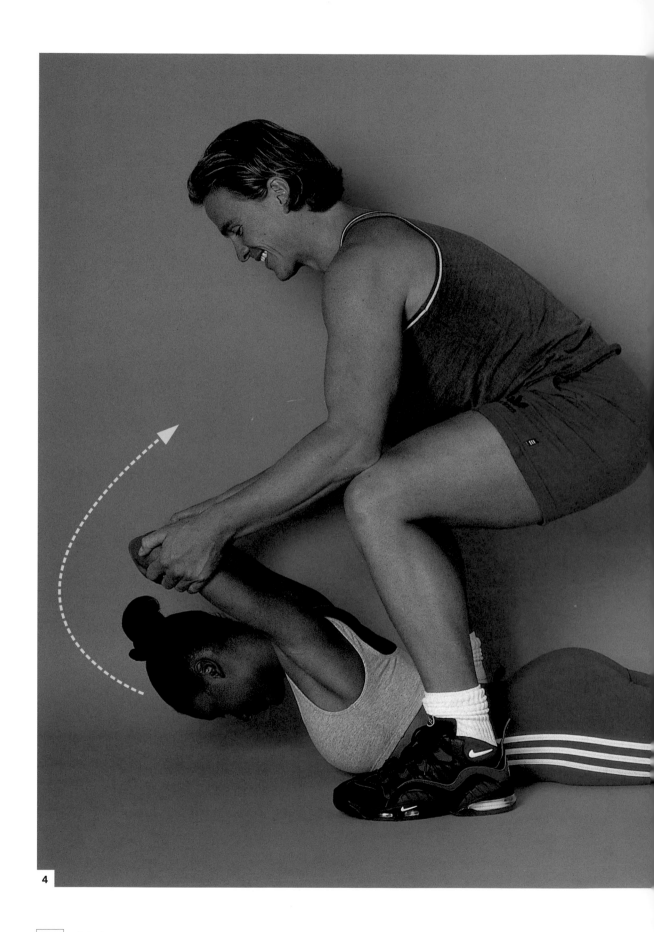

4

4. **COBRACATION**

This is a great stretch exercise for the arms, chest and shoulders, as well as helping to flex the lower back area, which is an important part to keep mobile.

THE STRETCHEE

The person being stretched lies face down on the floor and folds her arms, pressing her head through her arms to rest on the floor. Your partner will then pick you up by holding your arms and gently pulling them towards him.

You will feel a stretch around the shoulders and chest as your head falls forwards to hang below your arms and your arms are stretched back. You will also feel a bend in the lower back. All of these feelings should be pleasant. Nothing should be feeling as if it is being pulled too far. If you do experience any discomfort at all, then use the safety code words. Keep your breathing natural the whole time you are in the stretch position and think about relaxing your spine.

To get your body used to this stretch, you may need to try it once, release it, and then repeat it again.

THE LIFTER

Stand with feet apart and knees well bent as you reach down to lift your partner. Slide your hands gently beneath the upper arms, nearest the elbow joints, and once you have a good hold, gently lift her upper body upwards and back, towards you. Take care not to pinch the soft flesh of this area as you pick her up and arch her back slowly upwards. (Make sure you are checking that she is all right.)

When you are satisfied that she is comfortable, rest your bent arms on your knees. In this way, the position is stable and the weight of her body is taken by your legs, and not by your back.

Hold the stretch for just 15–20 seconds and then gently release her back to the floor. Be aware that her forehead will be the first thing to touch the floor, so lower her gently and with control. Gently massage her shoulders – this will help the muscles to recover.

Don't forget to swap roles so that the other person gets a chance to be stretched. There is no reason why two people of differing weights cannot perform this exercise perfectly well together – just bear in mind that, when the lighter person is doing the lifting, certain rules should be carefully observed (see box, left, 'Protect Your Back').

PROTECT YOUR BACK

Whenever you are lifting something heavy, you should protect your lower back by:

- *Always bending the knees and squatting down – to 90° only or just below – with the weight over the heels and the knees behind the toes.*
- *Pulling in on the stomach muscles and the pelvic floor muscles to support your internal organs.*
- *Pulling the object or person in close to you, with the strength in your arms.*
- *As you lift, pressing through the legs and buttocks to use the large muscles in these areas to lift the weight of the object or person. The upper body should be fairly upright.*
- *Remembering that you should never "hinge" from the back – always press through the legs.*

5. THE THIN EDGE OF THE WEDGE

This is a gentle stretch exercise that is excellent for stretching out and relaxing the shoulders and neck. It is especially good after a long, hard day or if you feel that your back is tight or have a headache.

THE PRESSEE

Have your partner sit comfortably in front of you, with her back straight and stomach pulled in. Now, using a very gentle touch and communicating all the time, work your way through the following sequence.

Place your right hand in front around the bottom of the throat, on the very uppermost part of the breastbone, and ease her back towards you, so that her weight is supported against your body. Now place the other hand on top of her head, pushing it gently downwards. You should feel that your two hands are pushing in opposite directions. One hand is keeping the spine tall while the other stretches the muscles at the back of the neck.

Now gently move your hand from the top of the head and, if possible, use it to grip her hair (not too tightly!) and pull her head into an upright position. Using the hair means that your partner doesn't have to use her neck muscles at all to lift her head, so that she can keep them as relaxed as possible.

Once upright, place your right hand on the left side of her head and your left hand on her left shoulder. Very, very gently, press down with the hand that is on the shoulder while the other hand guides the head over to the side (see photograph, opposite). Your partner will feel a stretch down the left side of her neck.

Do not hold this stretch for more than 10 seconds and, again, use the hair to lift the head back to an upright position. Now reverse the hand positions to repeat the stretch on the other side of her neck and finish the stretch by lifting her head so that it is upright.

Afterwards, you may wish to repeat the back-of-the-neck stretch once more and then gently place your fingers and thumbs across the back of the shoulders and massage this area very gently.

Finally, place the first two fingers of each of your hands on the sides of the neck and massage in small circles up the sides of the neck and down again.

THE STRETCHEE

The stretchee should really enjoy this exercise, which will take the tension out of her neck and the top of her shoulders. But do let your partner know if you feel that his touch is too hard or painful at any time. And don't forget to swap actions so you both get a chance to enjoy the feeling!

SAFETY NOTES

- *Don't press heavily on the side of her head. The head is very heavy – up to 12lb in weight – and although the neck muscles are used to supporting this weight they are still relatively thin and can easily be pulled. This is why mobilizing the neck is always a good idea (see Chapter 6).*
- *In fact, you don't need to exert pressure in this stretch at all. Simply keep the hand on the shoulder to stop it from lifting up and use your other hand to guide the head to one side.*

5

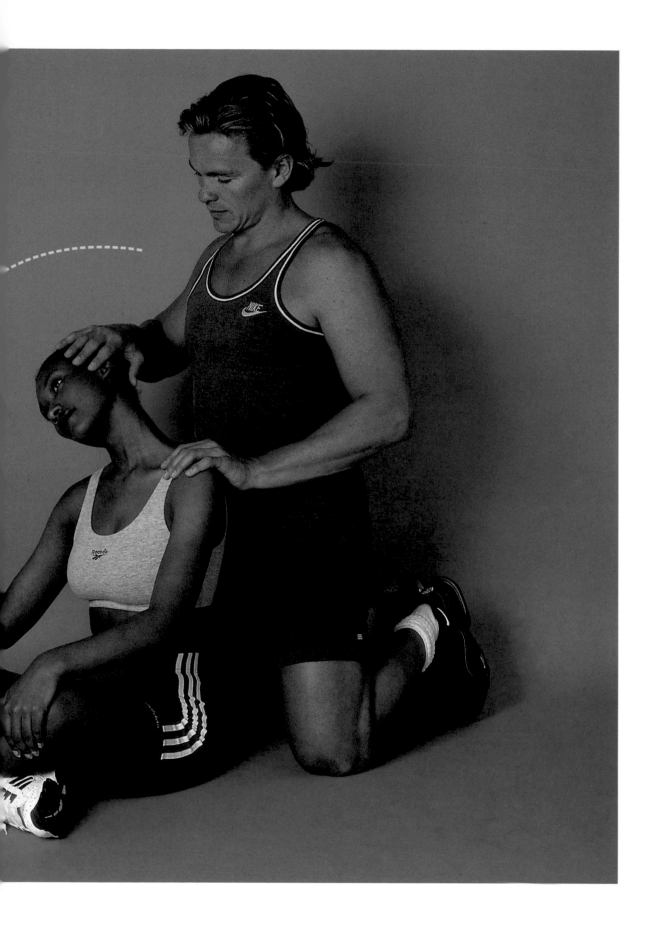

6. THE BACK RELEASER

This final partner sequence is not so much a stretch as a mobilizer and relaxer for the spine. One partner must give the complete weight of her legs to the other so that they can be supported and moved gently in any direction. This suspends any tension and weight that was pressing down on the lower back, bringing real relief. The process is so relaxing that it has to be felt to be believed and the only problem will be getting your partner off the floor to return the compliment!

THE PRESSEE

Stand above your partner, with your legs well bent in the squat position, and lift your partner's legs off the floor. Lift the feet only a foot or so off the ground and keep them at this height as you move them around.

Be careful not to hurt your back – a totally relaxed person has very heavy legs. Keep your knees bent with your stomach lifted for support and use the muscles in the arms to lift the legs.

NOW PERFORM THESE ACTIONS:

1. Keeping the feet level, lift the ankles gently up and down (only by about 5–8 cm).
2. Lift one leg and then the other, as if the legs were walking.
3. Bring the ankles together and move them in a circle, 2–3 times each way.
4. Gently shake the legs to check that your partner is relaxing her limbs fully.
5. Lift both feet and legs all the way up, walking your own feet forwards, until the soles of your partner's feet are facing the ceiling. At this point, you should feel the legs start to bend. Gently pull them straight and walk your feet back out again so that you lower her legs to a position that is just off the floor once more. Repeat this walk-in 2 or 3 times and, as you lower the legs for the last time, gently stretch the legs so that your partner experiences a mild traction (pull) as you relax her lower back.
6. Walk the legs all the way to one side, so your partner's body now forms an L shape (like a sideways bend); then repeat on the other

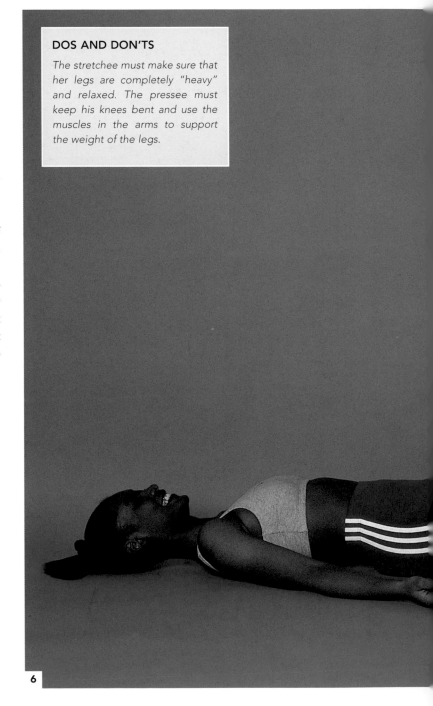

DOS AND DON'TS

The stretchee must make sure that her legs are completely "heavy" and relaxed. The pressee must keep his knees bent and use the muscles in the arms to support the weight of the legs.

6

side so that she also feels a stretch up the sides of the torso. Bring her legs gently back to centre.

7. To finish, hold both the ankles and shake them gently so that the shake goes up the length of her body before replacing her feet lightly on the floor.

8. Get your partner to roll over onto her side and then push herself up to a seated position to bring herself back slowly to a fully alert state.

Once she has recovered, she has to perform the same hard work for you!

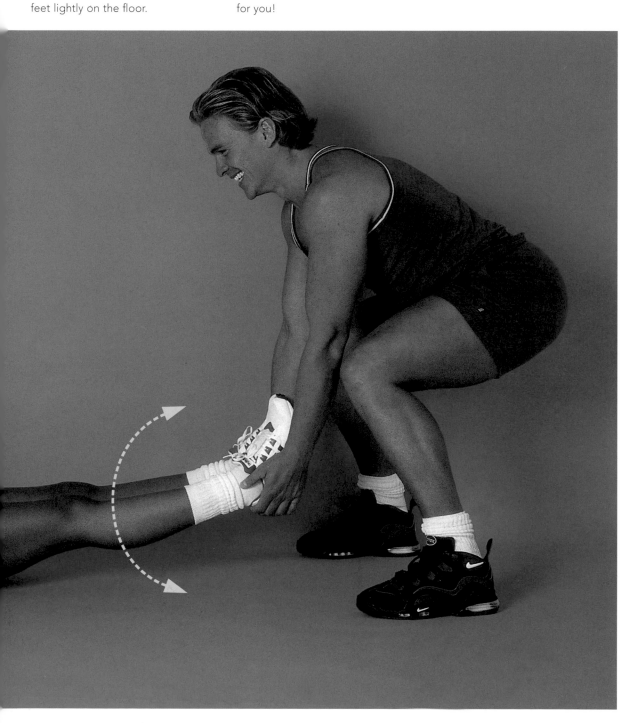

keep stretching

Stretching is important not only as part of a well-planned workout routine, but also as an activity by itself. Stretching sessions will keep you supple and feeling as if you can move without hindrance or pain. If you are exercising your body hard, and particularly if you are building up your muscles, then stretching is a must to keep your flexibility and range of movement. And as you get older, stretching should become an even more important aspect of maintaining flexibility in order to stay active.

GET MOVING

Stretching is also a good way to reintroduce the body to exercise and fitness. If you are recovering from an injury, for example, or even just a long period of inactivity, then a little stretching will get you flexible and moving again. Even those of us who are motivated to work out regularly can have periods where illness, work or family pressures disrupt our normal fitness regime, and stretching is one of the most pleasurable ways to reintroduce the body to movement.

Throughout this book you will find stretches that challenge the body as well as being pleasurable and helping to motivate you.

STRETCH AND CHILDBIRTH

After the birth of a baby is a good time to start a gentle stretching programme. You will find that it will revitalize the body and get it moving in ways that it has not been used to for quite a while. Over the following pages there is a selection of various antenatal and postnatal stretches designed to keep you supple all the way through your pregnancy and the months afterwards.

ILLNESSES AND INJURY

During your recovery after an injury or illness is another particularly good time to introduce some stretch sequences to your body. You may have been immobile for a while or a part of you may simply be stiff from lack of use, so turn to any of the stretches in this book that you feel will get that area moving.

PROBLEM SOLVING

This chapter also features stretches and mobilizers for problem areas – these are areas where many people experience some stiffness or lack of mobility. Pages 106–111 deal with stretches for the back, legs, neck and shoulders and suggest ways to mobilize and stretch these often stubborn areas.

If you haven't been moving athletically for quite some time, for whatever reason, then muscles and joints will tighten up and you will feel stiffer than you did when you were exercising regularly. This is because

muscles, ligaments and tendons all tighten slightly with lack of use and it takes regular "encouragement" sessions to get the synovial fluid lubricating the joints fully once again and the body accustomed to moving in particular ways. It also takes a certain amount of time for the mind to become used to not overreacting to the stretch reflex.

Always start with short, gentle sessions of stretch and mobilizing exercises to encourage and re-accustom the body to exercise. Bear in mind that when you first start, you may experience some stiffness the following day, so take things gradually. Along with stretching and mobilizing stiff areas, you may also like to try some gentle massage techniques to help relieve tension and discomfort in sore muscles. You will find some suggestions on the following page.

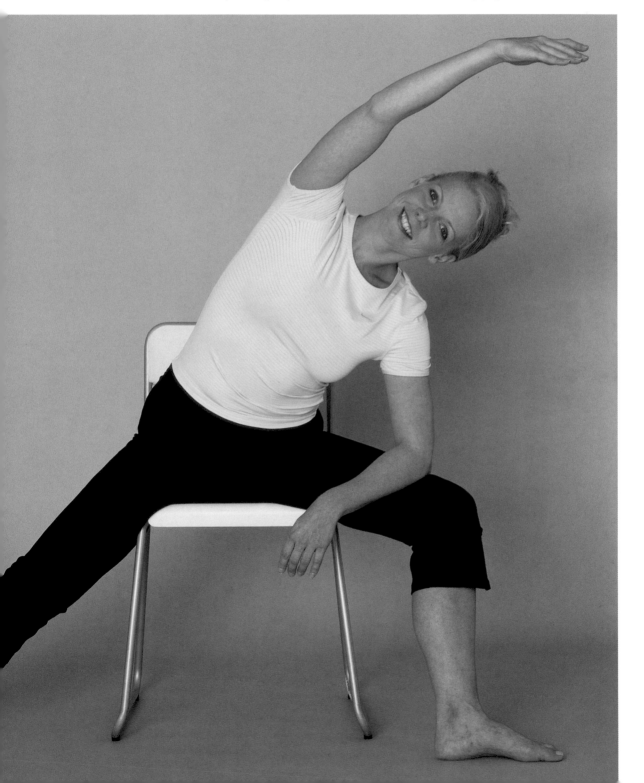

MASSAGE

Massage is an excellent way of helping the muscles of the body to relax. A full, all-over body massage should be given by a qualified therapist who will know the basic pressure points and ways of relieving them. Gently rubbing and cajoling a stiff area, however, is something anyone can do either for themselves or for their partner.

If you have stretched a certain area it can feel particularly good to gently rub, knead or pound the muscle, bringing blood back to the surface and creating some warmth. In the same way, if an area feels at all sore or stiff, lightly squeeze the muscles between thumb and fingers and knead along the line of the muscle to warm it and get it used to some movement.

Healthy muscles can easily be grasped and kneaded and should feel malleable and pliable without too many lumps or knots just below the surface. If you come across an area where your partner cries out with discomfort, you may need to spend some extra time on this region, gently pressing and kneading around the sore spot to release the tension. End your massage session with some light tapping (with cupped hands) or pounding to get the blood flowing through the area once again.

CRAMPS

When you are feeling stiff or under tension or stress you can sometimes experience cramps. Cramping is not fully understood, although it is thought to be due to a lack of calcium or possibly other minerals. What does seem certain, however, is that we are particularly prone to it at certain times of our lives –

SELF-HELP FOR CRAMP

If cramping does occur, try not to panic but immediately press with the heels of both hands on the area that you feel is in spasm. Pressing down on the contracted muscle will encourage it to flatten and relax its grip. As you feel the muscle release, you can then start to stretch the muscle, which will help to prevent the cramp from recurring immediately.

during periods of stress or during pregnancy, for example.

What happens with cramp is that the muscle contracts very strongly and stays contracted in a spasm, bringing sudden and alarming discomfort to the sufferer.

AIDING RECOVERY

Cramp can often leave the muscle feeling sore, so gentle rubbing, or even the application of some heat, can help the muscle recover. If you know you are prone to cramp, then regular stretching and massage of the area can really help. Pregnant women, for example, often experience cramp in their feet and calves at night, so in this case a gentle pre-sleep stretch could be a good idea. See page 105 for full directions.

INJURY

Injuries usually need proper medical attention and lots of rest. However, once you have taken professional advice, a gentle application of heat and cold can sometimes help to relieve any soreness or discomfort that may be there. If you have a sore or overworked muscle, then warming the area up is a must before you try to use it again.

A gentle warm-up (as detailed in Chapter 1) and gentle massage

around the area can help to bring blood to the sore area and prepare it for use once more.

There are also many products available on the market which warm the area. These are a good idea if used in moderation and as an extra – not as a substitute for proper warm-up exercises. Cold sprays are also available and these can help take the sting out of sore muscles after a workout. Do not use cold sprays before a workout, as these can numb the muscles and you need to be able to feel discomfort so that you know when you are overdoing things. Remember, pain is usually there for a reason and it is not advisable to ignore it or use a substance that might mask it.

At all times, do try and remember that stretching is a gradual process and that no amount of forcing, bouncing or stretching will stretch the muscles in one session. In fact, if you push things too far, you will be prone to overstretching and thus "pulling" or even tearing a muscle. Always try to work slowly and conscientiously towards your stretch goals, making the process a regular event in your life rather than a forced, one-off session.

A VISIT TO THE PHYSIOTHERAPIST

If you find you are very stiff or that, over the course of several weeks, your stretch ability is not improving, it may be worth a trip to the physiotherapist, just to check that there are no anatomical restrictions or other conditions that may be limiting you.

OTHER TIMES TO STRETCH

Remember, you can always find new opportunities to stretch if only you look for them! Stretch and mobilization exercises can help you throughout your week to keep the body ticking over and in good working order. In his book *Beirut Hostage*, John McCarthy wrote in detail of the basic exercise programme he instigated that helped to keep his spirits up when he was held in prolonged captivity.

AIRPLANE PLANS

A long period of enforced immobilization, of the type experienced during airplane flights, is a common situation where some gentle mobilization exercises will help to keep you feeling more alert and less jet-lagged at the end of your journey.

- For instance, from time to time throughout the flight, try rotating your ankles first one way and then the other. Repeat 5 or 6 times at one go.
- This simple routine will help to keep the ankles supple and help to encourage the blood flow through the legs – this can become sluggish when we sit in confined spaces for long periods of time.
- You can also repeat a similar action with the hands, rotating them at the wrists and stretching and bending the fingers.
- If you have enough room, try reaching up to the ceiling with both arms, stretching up as high as you can and lifting the weight upwards, off the spine.
- Breathe in deeply as you reach up and breathe out as you bring your arms down.

TV AND BOOK BENDING

Even while you are watching TV or reading a book, don't miss out on the opportunity to get a little stretching in!

- You could take both legs out to the side (see photo on page 37) and rest your elbows on the floor (if you can) and then rest your head on your hands as you watch your favourite TV show!
- Or you could sit with one leg bent and the other leg straight (see page 78) and lean forwards as you read your book, relaxing into the stretch on one leg.
- Don't forget to swap legs at the end of each chapter.

WATER WORKOUT

Even in the bath you can fit in the odd stretch! Your muscles will be nice and warm and relaxed so even though there isn't much room it could be a good place to stretch!

- Lie on your back and bend up one leg so that you can take hold of the ankle. Then try to straighten the leg towards you. As you get stretchier you should be able to pull the leg close to the wall behind your head!
- Always make sure your free foot is braced on the end of the bath so that you don't disappear under the water!

BUSMAN'S HOLIDAY

Even on a bus (or other mode of transport) if you find your back is feeling a little stiff from lack of movement or being curved for too long a period – give your body a break by placing your hands firmly on your knees. Now brace your arms as you press the top of your head towards the ceiling as far as you can while pressing your coccyx (the end-most part of the spine) down towards the seat. Breathe out as you press downwards and feel the spine release and extend. You can also do this exercise at home lying on your back with your legs at right angles over a bed or chair – this will really help stretch out the back.

Using these suggestions should give you the idea that you can use any activity as an opportunity to stretch. So don't miss out – mobilize!

antenatal
stretching

With a growing baby inside you, it is vital to keep supple. As you increase in size, there is obviously some loss of flexibility, while tiredness and other related problems tend to make you want to move around less. If you can manage some gentle stretch sessions in your working week, then this will help you to stay mobile for as long as possible and relieve some of the aches and pains of a long pregnancy.

SAFETY AND HORMONES

By the time the baby is beginning to show (around three to four months), a hormone called Relaxin is well established. Relaxin affects all the connective tissue of the body – for example, the joints, joint capsules, tendons and ligaments. The purpose of relaxin is to relax all the ligaments and muscles surrounding the pelvis in order to allow the baby to pass through the narrow opening.

In non-pregnant women, the tough connective tissue known as ligaments is supple but firm and will only stretch a small amount, to allow the joints to work within their natural range. In pregnancy, with the presence of Relaxin (more pronounced in second and third pregnancies), the affected ligaments may allow the joints to go beyond their normal range. This could cause damage to the joints or allow nerves to become trapped.

This means that great care must be taken when stretching during pregnancy. Only hold stretches for 8–10 seconds. This will ensure that there is no developmental stage to your stretches and that you keep well within your normal range.

GETTING COMFORTABLE

As your pregnancy progresses, you will find certain stretch positions very uncomfortable to get into. Lying on your front is, obviously, out of the question once your stomach begins to protrude, and lying on the back is not recommended after week 20 because it can cause faintness in some. Trying to take hold of a foot or leg or reaching forwards to pick something up can also be difficult.

The rule is this – use the positions that are most comfortable for you. Don't stay in any one position too long and keep the legs together as you change from pose to pose.

POSITION 1:

Sitting on the floor with your legs open enough to facilitate your bump, slowly walk the arms forwards until you feel a gentle stretch on the back of the legs and inner thighs. Hold for 8–10 seconds only and then walk your hands back in.
- Keep the back straight and the hands on the floor for support.
- Keep your breathing as natural and regular as possible.
- You can extend the feet, but don't over-point the toes as this could lead to cramp.

- Repeat this stretch 2–3 times.
- While you are in this position you should also remember to do your pelvic floor exercises!

POSITION 2:

Rest your hands on something solid like a chair and, keeping a slight bend in the knees, let the back straighten and the head fall through between the arms.
- You will feel a stretching and releasing sensation in the lower back, which is very relaxing for pregnant mums, where the weight of the foetus can bear down on the lower back curve if posture is not absolutely perfect.
- You may also feel a stretch in the shoulders, where the arms are extended.
- Don't allow the stomach to sag downwards in this position and the back to arch; keep the back as straight, and as supported by the stomach muscles, as possible.
- Keep breathing regularly throughout and only hold the position for 8–10 seconds, walking your feet back in and curling up through the body to come out of the stretch.

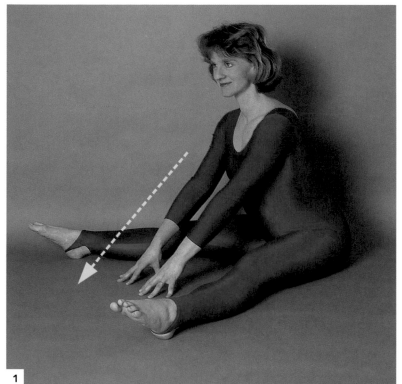

1

TOWEL TIP

Using a towel can sometimes be a help; perhaps by wrapping it around your foot or leg when you cannot reach very far. Always try to keep your back straight and remember that you can still pull in on the stomach muscles, even if they are stretched beyond all recognition!

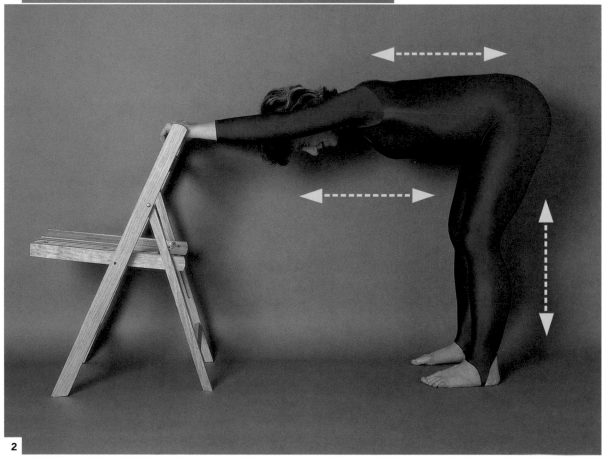

2

postnatal
stretching

Congratulations! Now that you have had your baby, you can start to remobilize the areas of your body that have become unaccustomed to moving. It is generally accepted that women can begin to work out properly after they have had their six-week check-up from the doctor.

As well as the stretches featured here, you can also begin to include the warm-up section (see Chapter 1) in your regime, as well as any of the beginners' stretches, to start challenging your whole body. Just remember to take it easy, and work slowly over the next three months to increase your general level of fitness – you should not feel any pain.

AROUND THE MIDDLE

One of the principal areas of the body that suffers from inactivity during pregnancy is the waist and middle torso. As the baby grew, your waist will have thickened and the chances are you have not done too much side bending and hip wiggling for the last few months. Now is the time to start! Side bends and revolving the hips can awaken the side of the torso and the oblique abdominal muscles, preparing them for the toning and strengthening exercises that you should include in your postnatal workout.

POSITION 1:

Stand up straight with your knees slightly bent and hips tucked under. Remember to pull in strongly on the stomach and to lift the back now that you no longer have your bump to worry about!

With hands on your hips, slowly circle the hips anticlockwise, push-ing the hips as far in each direction as you can. Then circle back the other way to make one complete rotation.

- Repeat 6–7 times in each direction.
- Then wiggle the hips from side to side while bending the knees and repeat the circles once more.

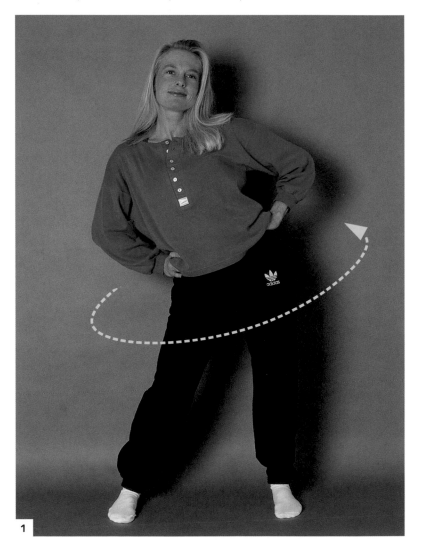

1

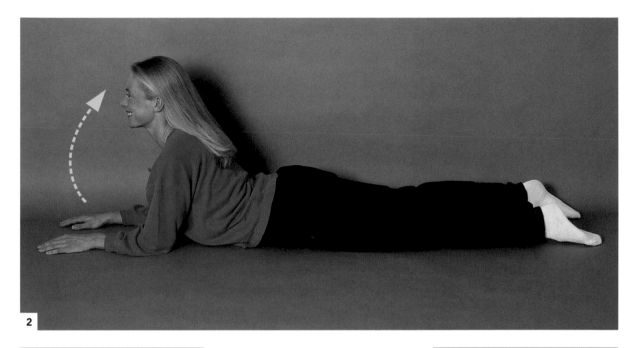

2

CRAMP AND PREGNANCY

Pregnant women can be prone to cramp, and this problem may continue after the birth, too. Cramping often occurs at night or on waking, and often in the feet and legs. Try practising the following stretch before you go to sleep, or when you first wake:

- *Stand with one hand resting against a wall and place one foot in front of the other. Now take all your weight onto the back foot (the other foot is still resting on the floor). Bend both knees gently until you feel a stretch at the back of the back leg. You can hold this stretch for up to 20 seconds and then straighten the legs to release. Repeat with the other leg in front. This position will help to stretch the lower calf muscle and the Achilles tendon area.*
- *Alternatively, standing on a low stair and letting the heels of both feet rest over the edge of the stair will also stretch out the calves. Keep the back straight and the abdominals pulled in.*

POSITION 2:

Something else you won't have done for a long time is lying on your tummy – so start trying it now. If you have had a caesarean, you may feel quite sore across the stomach, so approach this stretch very gently. If the exercise pulls too much and feels uncomfortable, then leave it till a later date.

Once you are used to taking weight on your stomach once more, try the following exercise: place your elbows underneath yourself and slowly lift your head and shoulders off the floor.

- This stretches the abdominals and mobilizes the lower back.

It is very important to look after your back post-natally – this is an area that is still much-affected by the Relaxin hormone and the strain of carrying and bearing a child makes it very unstable. A gentle mobilizing of the back area, like the stretch illustrated above, will help, along with some strengthening work.

SAFETY NOTES

The Relaxin hormone (see page 102) may still be present after you have given birth. It can stay in the body for at least five months if you are breastfeeding, so be aware that any stretching you do in the first six months must be done carefully and should not include the developmental stage.

problem
areas

LEGS

When you are trying to stretch, or even simply carrying out everyday actions, you may find that one area is often stiffer than others and stiff legs is a common problem. Is lifting your leg to get over a fence difficult? Or is sitting up straight with both legs stretched out in front of you un-comfortable? This may be due to stiffness in the back of the legs (the hamstrings) or the groin area (adductor muscles). If you do experience stiffness in these areas, it is worth spending extra time doing a variety of stretches to increase your flexibility and rid yourself of any limitations in your daily movements.

POSITION 1:

One of the best ways to develop your stretch is to adopt a position in which you can relax and so allow the muscles to start to lengthen. This position develops your groin stretch.

Lie on the floor with your backside as near the wall as you can manage and allow the legs to open equally to either side. Rest the legs fully against the wall and relax.

- The weight of your legs will start to stretch the muscles of the inner thighs as you maintain t his position and you will feel a powerful but gradual stretch as you relax completely.
- Don't stay in this position for too long – 1–2 minutes is enough time – and use your hands to push your legs together and then roll out of the stretch.
- Gently knead or rub your inner thigh muscles to relieve them from the stretch, then stand up and shake the legs out.

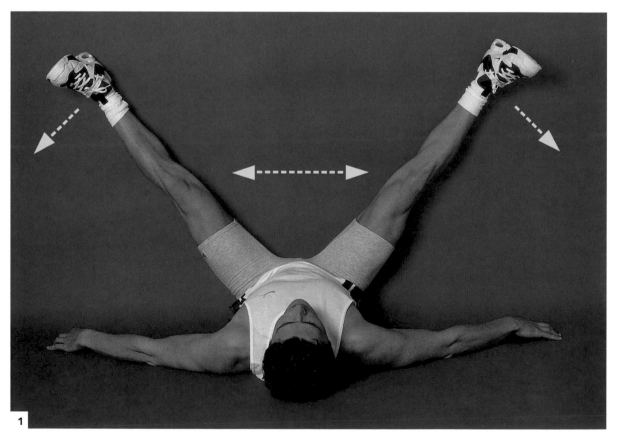

1

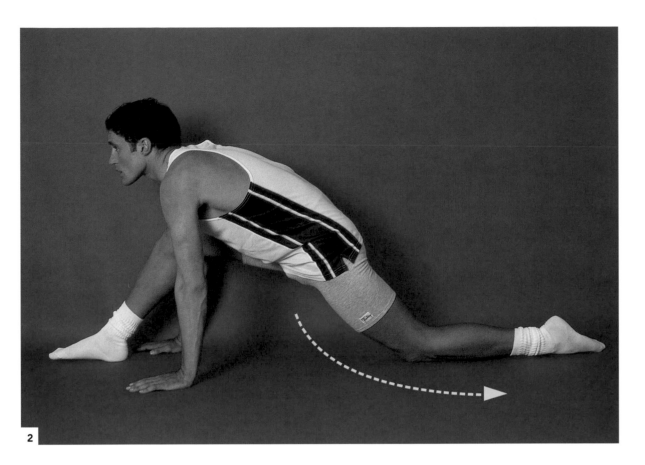

2

POSITION 2:

The splits stretch position works on enhancing flexibility not just in the groin area but also on the back of the legs and the front of the thighs. You might think that the splits is beyond your abilities, but if you approach the position gradually and attempt it regularly, you will notice the groin getting nearer and nearer to the floor over the weeks to come. Try this with caution, and stop if you feel any pain.

The easiest and safest way to get into splits is outlined here:

• Start in the lunge position (page 38) and, with hands on the floor, gently press the groin several times towards the floor. Now drop the knee of the back leg to the floor and place both hands on the front knee. Press the hips forward several times – so that you feel a

stretch along the front of the thigh (of the back leg).

• Repeat 2 or 3 times, pressing slightly further each time.

• Now tuck the back foot flat (so that the top of the foot is resting on the floor). With hands on the floor for support, slowly slide the back foot away from the front leg, behind you, and let it take you down into the splits. Don't move the front leg at all but simply slide the back leg away from you as far as it is comfortable to do.

• Hold for 10 seconds before releasing, shaking the legs out and then trying the same on the other side.

• If you do this every day for a period of 2 weeks you will be closer to the ground by at least a foot at the end of that time.

Other ways to stretch the back of the legs and groin area include:

• Placing one foot on a higher surface – for example, on a chair or table – and leaning forwards over the straight leg. You will feel the stretch in the back of the raised leg.

• You can also place the leg in the same position but at the side of you, so that, as you lean over, you will feel the stretch in the side of the torso as well as the inner thigh.

• Once you have a leg raised on something stable, you can even lean over forwards, taking your hands onto the floor or letting them hang either side of the leg. In this way you will feel the stretch in the groin and the back of the supporting leg.

BACK

Common back problems range from serious slipped discs and paralysis to constant aches and pains that remain unexplained but are nevertheless very tiresome. A lot of back problems, however, originate from misuse or lack of use of that area – especially bad posture.

The spine is actually designed to curve, bend and extend freely in all directions. It does not respond well to constant pressure from bad posture (slumping or leaning backwards on the lower back), stiffness from being forced and held in one position all the time (for instance if someone is always bent over a desk) or general inactivity.

Physiotherapists often remark that if people did some more exercise, strengthening and flexing the spinal area, then there would be far fewer back problems. If you develop a sore back or a nagging backache, try some gentle limbering exercises while you are waiting for an appointment with your doctor (take care, and stop if the stretches cause pain). These may well solve the problem and ease the tensions before you even make it to the doctor's surgery!

POSITION 1:

One very relaxing back stretch is to lie on your back and bring the knees up towards your chest. Take your hands out to the side and rest them on the floor for balance. Now, keeping the knees together, tip the legs over to one side and rest them completely on the floor.

- Stay in this position for up to a minute and then swing the legs to the other side and rest there.

- This gently twists the spine and allows tension to seep away.

There are many variations on this stretch: you can swing one knee over with the other knee following, for example, which opens the hips out as you swing from side to side. You can also have one leg straight and take just one knee across the body towards the opposite side, which gives a slightly more intense twist in the spine. The best approach is to experiment a little to see which position feels more comfortable for you and brings the most relief.

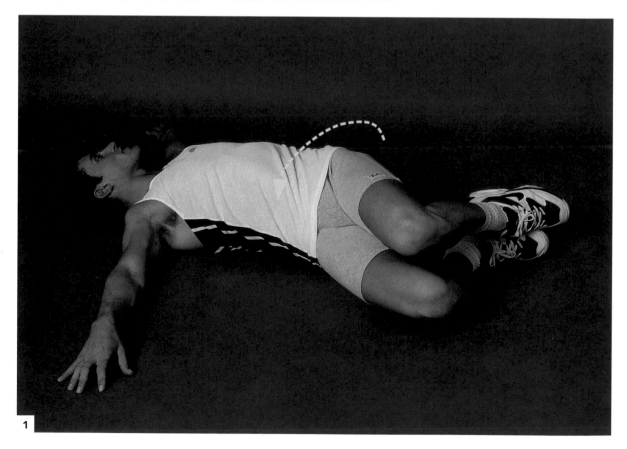

1

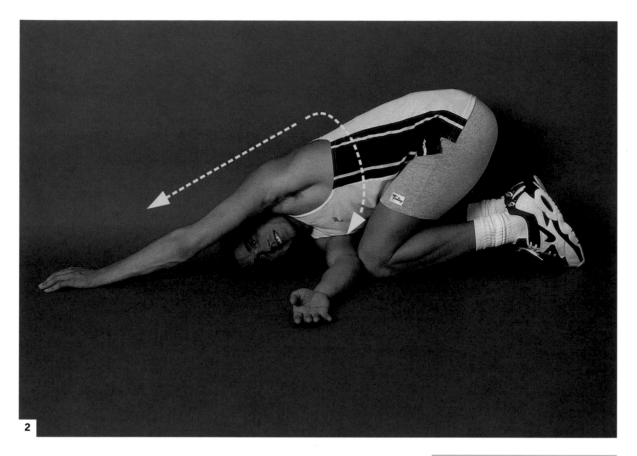

2

POSITION 2:

This is a stretch specifically intended for the upper back.

Start by kneeling with both arms outstretched and resting on the floor. Rest your forehead on the floor and feel the release in your back as you maintain this pose for a while. Now thread one arm underneath and across the body and rest the side of your head on the floor.

• You will feel a relaxing stretch across the upper back.

• Hold this position for up to 1 minute and then repeat the exercise on the other side.

Some other beneficial ways to stretch the back include: lying on your back and bringing the feet into your chest; pressing the soles of the feet together; or even raising the legs up over the body so that only

the shoulders remain on the floor. You will feel this stretch all along your back as well as through the back of the legs.

Move into and out of these positions slowly and only take them as far as is comfortable for you. Listen to your body.

KNOW YOURSELF

Bear in mind that flexibility varies tremendously from person to person, and some stretches will feel more pleasurable or challenging than others. In addition, you may find that you feel the stretch in a slightly different area to the one mentioned. This does not necessarily mean you are doing it incorrectly in any way, but that the tightness/elasticity in the muscles gives rise to different sensations in different places. As long as you are not in pain, you are probably doing the position correctly.

NECK AND SHOULDERS

The shoulders and neck area are often in need of regular stretching. The smallish neck muscles not only support a heavy skull but also carry a lot of our general tension. It is always a good idea to get someone to massage this area on a regular basis, as this can help to alleviate and prevent strain. Learning how to stretch the head and neck area for yourself as a form of self-massage will also help.

POSITION 1:

Start by sitting cross-legged with the back straight, and then place both your hands on the back of your head. Lift your elbows out to the side and press the head forwards as far as you can go.

- Don't allow the back to curve or the stomach to sag; the torso should be held fairly straight and lifted. Curve just from the base of the neck.
- As you hold this pose, you will feel the back of the neck stretching out.
- Hold for 10–15 seconds.

You can release the tension even further by keeping one hand on the top of your head and then using the first finger and thumb of the other hand to press lightly up the sides of the neck. Press the fingers in firmly, right up into the hair, and then down again. This will help to release the soreness and tension that builds up in the back of the neck and across the shoulders.

POSITION 2:

Now, sitting up straight with your abdominals lifted, tilt your head so that your left ear moves towards your left shoulder. Make sure that the shoulder is not lifted but is pressed down. Hold this for a few seconds and then take your left hand and gently place it on the side of your head to increase the stretch.

- Hold for 15 seconds then remove your hand and bring the head upright and then repeat on the other side.
- This sequence will help to stretch and relieve the muscles at the side of the neck.

To continue this exercise, take the head forwards again and rest your chin on your chest. Use the fingers

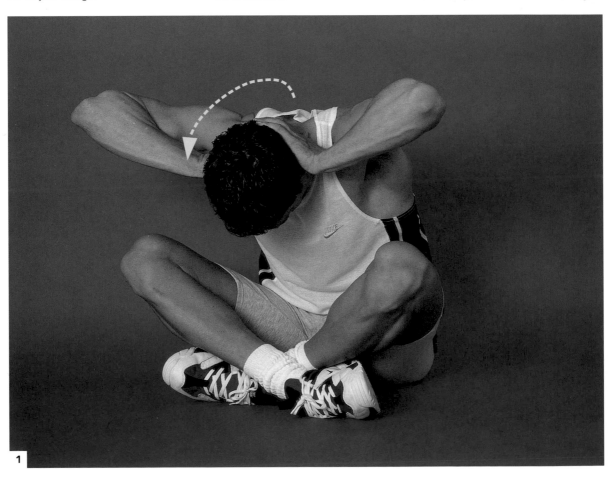

1

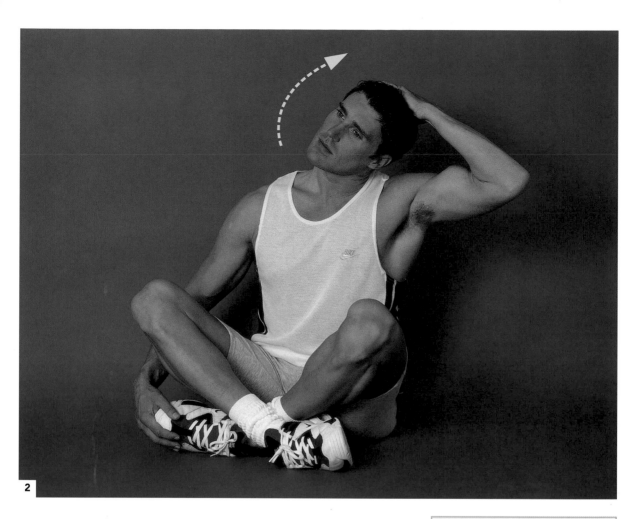

2

of both hands to press at intervals along the sides of the neck, right out to the top of the shoulders and back again. If you feel a particularly sore area, keep your fingers on it and massage in a circular motion to help release any knotted tension.

• This will help release tension and stiffness along the trapezius muscle which runs across the shoulders and down the back (see pages 10–11).

HEAD ROLLS

Doing headrolls is another effective way to release the neck from tension and promote mobility in the neck and shoulder region. There is some controversy, however, concerning just how safe it is to drop the head

backwards. It is possible that doing this could lead to trapped nerves, but it should be remembered that the head does need to make this action naturally from time to time, so it is better to practise it properly than to avoid it completely and risk becoming stiff as a result.

Make sure you circle your head with control (don't swing or fling it), slowly and smoothly. Start by taking the head forwards (the chin to chest) and then roll it around to the side and gently to the back and around to the other side. Then repeat, taking the head round in the other direction. Perform 4 or 5 head rolls until the "clicks" and "grinds" heard in the neck disappear.

SPOT CHECK

If you know that you have a tendency to hold strain and tension in your neck area, then try to check every so often during the day whether tension is building up here, especially if you are having a stressful time. Make sure your shoulders aren't hunched towards your ears – press them down, squeezing the shoulder blades together at your back. This quick stretch exercise is a great instant tension-reliever.

7 stretch for **relaxation**

Stretching isn't just a way of increasing your fitness potential – it is also a highly pleasurable aid to relaxation. Stretching can release tension from shortened and over-stressed muscles and in this chapter you will find stretch positions that will let all kinds of tensions seep out of your mind and body.

If the body is held in rigid stances throughout the day, then placing it in the opposite position and allowing it to rest there can help the muscles "let go" and relax. After sitting down for a long time, for example, stretching can be just as relaxing as a hot bath. Perhaps you have had a long flight on an aeroplane or have been seated for hours at a conference – whatever the circumstances, stretching is one of the best ways to improve the circulation gently and loosen up the stiff areas, reawakening the body and preventing stiffness and soreness from setting in.

In the previous chapter, you will have seen the stretches for problem areas – all of which help relieve tension in these vulnerable places. Even stretching in the bath or while watching T.V. will increase your sense of relaxation and well-being. Stretch positions are usually better than simply lying flat out, because only slightly twisted positions can often give full relief to such areas as the upper back or buttocks.

THE DOUBLE QUAD

Try, for example, adopting the position shown in the photograph.

Lie on your front and reach behind you to take hold of both your ankles. Grasp them firmly and then try to relax into the position. You will feel the stretch mainly on both upper thighs and across the hips. You will find that this is a particularly great way of relaxing the legs if you have been pounding the streets or going up and down stairs.

Let your hips sink down towards the floor and turn your head to the side or else rest your forehead on the floor if this is more comfortable. Keep your breathing regular and relaxed and enjoy the sensation of your leg muscles slowly extending and releasing their grip.

To come out of the stretch, release your hold on the ankles, and then use your hands to push yourself back onto all fours; massage the front of the thighs gently.

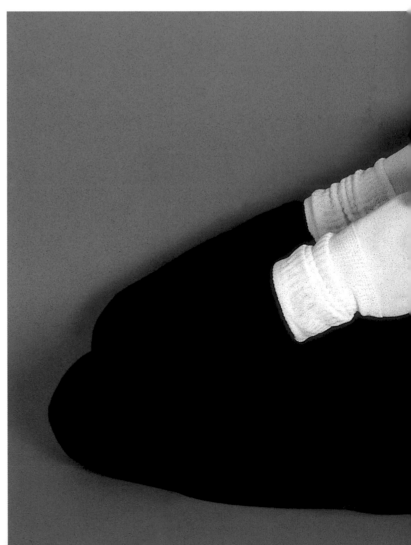

GOING WITH THE FLOW

In this chapter you will also find some stretch routines that flow together. The purpose of these is to use your stretch as a way of moving smoothly and gently, in a way that will bring relaxation and pleasure. Once you have performed these routines several times, you will come to know them off by heart and you can do them as little de-stress sessions during your day or just as a way of stretching out. You can also perform them with different goals in mind and with different music in the background, to really create a very specific mood-matching atmosphere. As you keep repeating these routines, you will be able to discover different ways to make the most of them. So, get stretching and start relaxing!

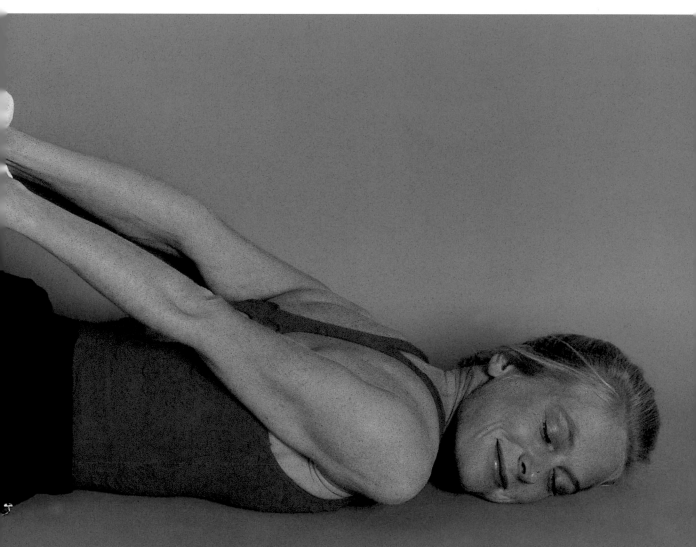

STRETCH TO RELAX

Many types of relaxation technique use tensing and stretching as a way to bring mind and body together and so aid total relaxation. Yoga uses many stretching postures that emphasize breathing and holding, so that the mind and body work in harmony. Dance, t'ai chi, and many other types of martial arts use stretching and relaxation side by side. When approaching your re-laxation stretches, try to focus your mind on what your body is feeling. In this way you will achieve a clearness of mind and a relaxation of the body that will refresh you completely.

STRETCH OUT

Try, for example, just lying flat on the floor on your back with your arms above your head. Now stretch out the whole body as far as you possibly can. Extend the legs from the hip joints and press right down through the knees to the toes. Feel your head and neck extending in the opposite direction and then imagine the spaces between each vertebra increasing as you stretch. You are growing longer!

Now release the stretch and just allow the body to sink back into the floor. Start to take note of which body areas are touching the floor and pressing down into it. Which limbs or part of limbs remain raised off the floor? Think through your entire body, starting at the head, and make sure that every part that could rest its weight on the floor is, in fact, doing so.

Finally, take note again where your body touches the floor, working through bit by bit, and use the parts that touch as a focus for tension to disappear. Imagine that wherever the body touches the floor there is a

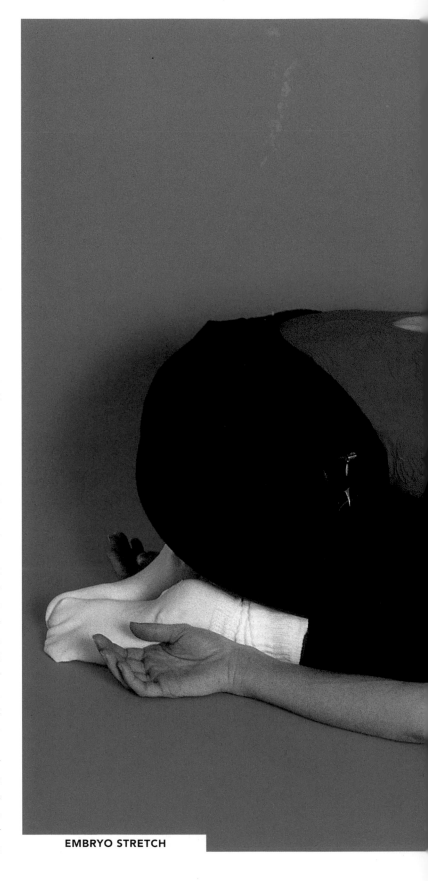

EMBRYO STRETCH

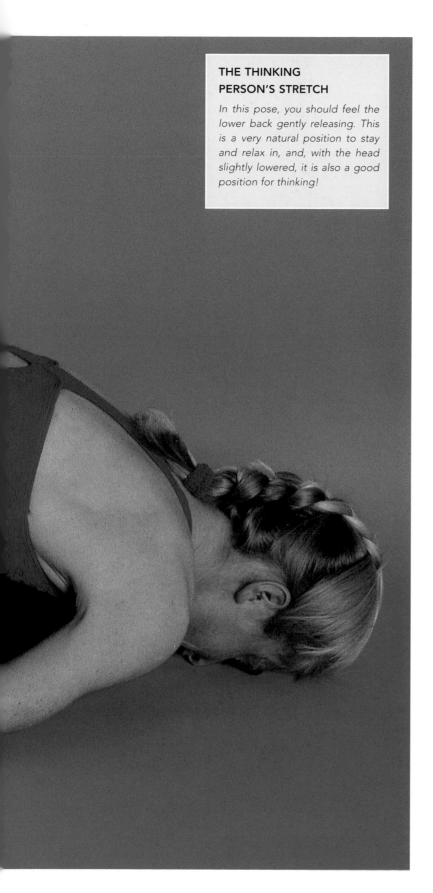

deep well below that draws out
tension from the muscles and drains
it into and beneath the floor. Repeat
the stretch one more time and relax
again afterwards.

EMBRYO STRETCH

This is a great relaxation position to
try when you are feeling tired out
and, although it may not appear so,
it will stretch and relieve your lower
back. Start by kneeling low on the
knees and stretch your arms out in
front of you and rest the flat of the
hands and the forehead on the floor.
Your bottom should be nearly on
your heels. Maintain this stretch for
a while – here you will benefit from a
stretch in the shoulders and arms as
well as the lower and upper back.

Now gently bring your hands
around to the sides of the body and
rest here. This subtly changes the
weight of the stretch, relaxing the
lower back even further and putting
slightly more weight on the forehead, which is also a good release
point for tension.

THE PRAWN STRETCH

To get into the pose shown in the photograph below, take the following steps. Lie on your back with both arms out to the sides and legs straight down, relaxed on the floor. Lift your right leg up to the ceiling and then, keeping it as straight as possible, tilt the leg all the way over, so that your foot touches the opposite (left) hand. To accomplish this, the hips will have to tilt with you. Hold this stretch for 10–20 seconds to feel it across the back and underneath the leg.

Now bend up the leg underneath (which at present is straight) and try and grasp its toes with your free hand. This may sound strange but once you are in position you can start to relax into it and will find that it is a very effective stretch.

Try to pull your two hands away from each other, gently, so that your two legs are being pulled in opposite directions. You should feel the stretch up the back of the top leg and across the groin and back, as well as in the front thigh of the leg underneath. Try to stay in this position for 20–30 seconds, breathing easily and concentrating on letting the muscles relax into position and into the floor. Gently release your hold on both feet and slowly bring the legs back to their original position and rest briefly. Repeat on the other side.

After you have stretched both sides, hug your knees into your chest and rock gently from side to side to relax the hips and legs.

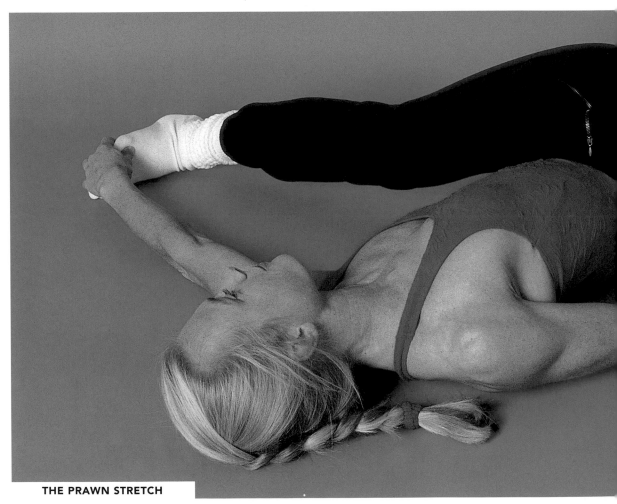

THE PRAWN STRETCH

stretching
for life

TEACHING CHILDREN

An experienced teacher will never push a child beyond his or her natural limits, at any age. Instead, the teacher should work with the natural mobility children have in order to bring co-ordination and fluidity to their movements. In this way, patterns of movement and activity will become established that could last a lifetime.

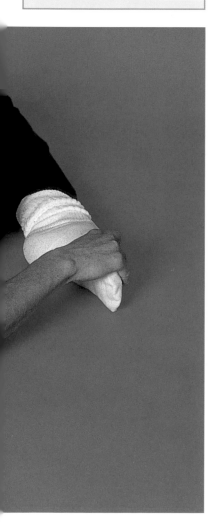

Remember that you are never too young or too old to start stretching and keeping limber. As long as your programme of stretches is tailored to your needs and your body at each stage of life, and you exercise regularly, then you should not suffer any injuries. All there should be is increased flexibility and pleasure in your movement.

AN EARLY START

If you have children, encourage them to run around and make as much use of their limbs as possible. Gymnastic and dance classes are always a good idea to introduce your child to some basic strength and flexibility work at an early age. The earlier children learn some simple co-ordinating movements the better, and if they can learn to manipulate their own body weight, they will develop natural strength and agility that may help to prevent accidents and stand them in good stead for the rest of their lives.

Above all else, early movement should be a source of pleasure and enjoyment for children, who will then, hopefully, continue with the habit as they grow.

LATER LIFE

In the later years of life, stretching exercises are one of the best forms of preventive medicine. They keep the joints mobile and help with balance and co-ordination as you get older. If you have been inactive

for a long time, always check with your doctor before starting any kind of exercise programme and then start gradually and build up to longer, more energetic, sessions as you start to feel the benefits.

As you are trying the exercises in this book, move into them all carefully and do not, under any circumstances, force anything. The stretch should feel challenging, but comfortable. The real test is whether or not the stretch is comfortable enough for you to maintain it for up to 30 seconds if you had to. If you feel anything pulling or being twisted, then stop and move onto another stretch. Keep your stretches varied and make sure that they cover all the areas of your body.

Try some swimming and walking to complement your stretching programme and only do what is comfortable for you. Switch to slightly different moves if certain stretches trouble you. But above all, remember that age is not a barrier and we can benefit at all ages from regular, easy movement.

flexibility
life-plan

IN YOUR 20s

You're probably single and enjoying the freedom from studies and parents. You may have a big group of friends and, if you're working, some regular money for the first time. But this may also be the first time you are away from organized exercise (in school or college); you may also suddenly have a much more sedentary life if you're sitting in an office for long hours.

HOW DO YOU FEEL ABOUT EXERCISE?

You may a feel a little de-motivated – there are so many other things to deal with – but you mustn't give up. Build it into your working life as quickly as you can. Exercise and keeping flexible should be fun in your 20s, a social event as well as a health necessity. Make sure your programme includes strength work, something that gets you running about a lot – and stretching!

WHAT'S YOUR BODY DOING?

Heart and lung capacity (used in aerobic exercise) start to decline once you hit 25 – unless you work out regularly. Your bones reach their peak mass during your early 20s; you can maximize density with weight-bearing exercises (where you use your own body weight to strengthen your muscles, as in press-ups or squat thrusts), making bones stronger and helping to prevent osteoporosis later in life. You still burn calories at a good rate, so make the most of that to reach your target weight by the age of 30.

STRETCH:

All areas of the body. Try to do at least 5–10 minutes, three times a week. Use all types of stretching methods (as described in this book) and have fun with it. Try attending stretching workshops or dance programmes that include flexibility workouts.

IN YOUR 30s

There is even more going on! You may be married, having children, forging busy careers. There never seems to be enough time. Beware – this is where the rot can really set in if you're not careful.

HOW DO YOU FEEL ABOUT EXERCISE?

Guilty probably, unless you've kept it going since your 20s. You'd like to work out, but when you have the time you're too tired. You view exercise as a weapon to fight that getting-old feeling, but also as a chore.

WHAT'S YOUR BODY DOING?

Your aerobic capacity is on the decline, so use it before you lose it. You are burning calories more slowly, so weight may be creeping on and affecting flexibility. You have already reached peak muscle mass, and will lose it unless you exercise. Your muscles are now less elastic and without regular stretching will become more prone to injury. If you have had children, your abdominal muscles may be slack and you may start to suffer from backache.

STRETCH:

For 10 minutes each day (see the programmes in Chapter 3) and include specific stretches for any particularly stiff areas (see Chapter 6). Include all types of stretches in your programme. Try some yoga or martial arts for a different kind of stretch.

IN YOUR 40s

Job and family life have probably settled into some kind of routine. Children can amuse themselves a bit more and you may have a little more time to yourself. Your child-bearing years are waning and you may feel the need for a new focus in life.

HOW DO YOU FEEL ABOUT EXERCISE?

Perhaps you would feel out of place in an aerobics class (where the average age is about 25). You may be carrying some extra weight and feel slower and more easily breathless. But don't despair – it's not too late to establish good habits and a regular regime. Starting now can improve your fitness later and will help blood flow, enhancing skin and muscle tone and even reversing some of the signs of ageing.

WHAT'S YOUR BODY DOING?

Arms and breasts can start to sag without muscle toning exercises and lung capacity declines without regular aerobic work. Fat cells are stored on bottom, stomach and thighs, while a dramatic reduction in muscle protein means you can lose a lot of speed and strength if you don't work to keep it. You may feel stiffer if you haven't been doing your flexibility homework and might be experiencing the first signs of the menopause.

STRETCH:

Everywhere you can, but keep it comfortable and avoid pushing or too many developmental stretches. Try to do 5–10 minutes as least twice a week. Concentrate on getting back any flexibility you feel you might have lost. Use this book to help you identify your stiff areas and then how to improve them and experiment with t'ai chi, gentle yoga classes and relaxation techniques.

IN YOUR 50s AND 60s

The children have left home so you have time for new interests. The menopause may have left you feeling a need to rethink your role in life.

HOW DO YOU FEEL ABOUT EXERCISE?

You know it's important but you might have forgotten how or where to start!

WHAT'S YOUR BODY DOING?

You're burning calories more slowly, so you need to eat less or opt for many more low-fat options in order to stay the same weight. You may feel weaker, particularly in the upper body, and bone mass is lost rapidly, with a real risk of osteoporosis – weight-bearing exercise where you use your own body weight to strengthen your muscles or work with dumbbells will help. Your joints will be stiffer and you will feel less flexible.

STRETCH:

All parts of the body. Check everyday flexibility – can you reach up and down your back? Are you happy twisting right around to see behind you in the car? If the answer is no, then work on these areas first (see Chapters 1 & 2). Try to do at least 5–10 minutes three times a week and build up from there. Don't worry about too many developmental stretches; keep your routines comfortable and try some of the moving routines in this chapter for fun. Also try: stretches for relaxation (see this chapter) and brisk walking and swimming. Don't forget the benefits of massage as a way of rediscovering your muscles and the pleasure of relieving them.

"wake up!"

This stretch routine is great for waking up in the morning – whatever age you are. It will get the blood flowing, the limbs moving and help you throw off that lingering sleepy feeling. If it appeals, you can do this to your favourite piece of music; make it rousing and upbeat if you have a busy morning ahead or just inspiring to set you up for the day.

FEEL THE STRETCH

Hold each position long enough to feel the stretch in each muscle and then carry on moving onto the next movement. In this way you will start to memorize the routine so that you can perform it as a whole piece of choreography. Once you have become familiar with it (and the accompanying music), you can then start to give different emphasis to different parts. For instance, you might want to prolong the reach-up at the beginning as you reach up high and fill your lungs with morning air. Or you might want to stay in position 3 for longer to feel the legs really stretching out.

Whichever way you do it, put some energy and emotion into your stretches. Try to feel the music in your movement and fill the notes with long, sustained reaches of your limbs. Use your eyes to follow your hand or foot as it extends so that you are sending energy out beyond your body and across the room.

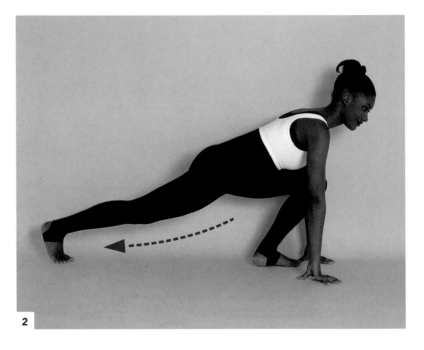

2

POSITION 1:

- Reach both hands to the ceiling and stretch up through the spine as high as you can.
- Feel the pull through the spine and imagine the spaces between the vertebrae widening. Let the reach of your arms nearly pull you onto your toes.
- This stretches the spine all the way through to the neck.
- Let the hands start to arch you backwards so that you bend the spine gently. Keep the feeling of lift as you arch high.
- Only arch backwards as far as feels comfortable and keep the head supported rather then dropping it right back.
- This flexes the spine, particularly the lower back area and the neck.

POSITION 2:

- From the arch position, stretch your arms to the sides as you bring them back down. Squeeze shoulder blades together.
- Sweep the right arm up and across your chest so that it leads the way as your shoulders twist to the left, turning your whole body to form a left-facing, sideways pose.
- Sink into a lunge, keeping your back leg as straight as possible, and take both hands and body over your front knee.
- Feel the stretch in the groin as you lower into the lunge. Keep the front knee in line with the toe and don't collapse the upper body over the leg. Hold to increase the stretch. This stretches the shoulders, chest, groin and legs.

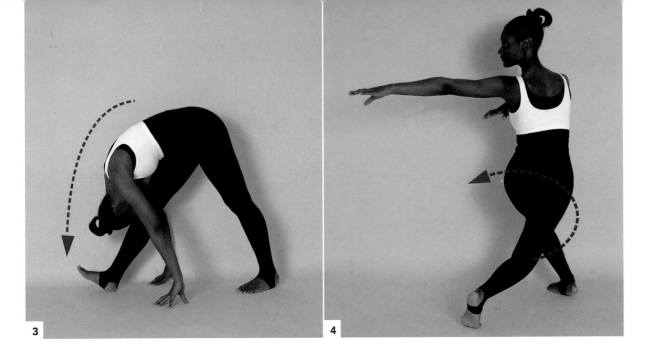

3

4

POSITION 3:

- From your lunge position, push the front knee to straighten the leg. Feel the back of the leg and straighten only as much as is bearable. Press the head towards the knee and then finally lift the front toes.
- You will feel a pull in the back of the legs as you perform this, so hold only for as long as you are comfortable and don't worry if you cannot get your leg straight the first time you try.

- Flex the foot and bring the toes towards you to increase the effect of the stretch.
- This stretches the back of the legs and ankles.

POSITION 4:

- To complete this sequence, bend the front leg back into a lunge. Now twist the body towards your front leg, and keep on twisting round in this direction, laying your back leg onto the floor. With your front leg bent, this will bring you into a sitting twist.

POSITIONS 5 AND 6:

- Continue the twisting motion in the upper body to finish with the head and shoulders twisted even further round than the hips.
- Curl in tightly to make your curl as compact as you possibly can and, with the final twist, feel the stretch in the waist. This stretches the torso and you will also feel it in the hips and legs.
- Come up to a standing position and repeat the sequence on the other side – you should now be wide awake!

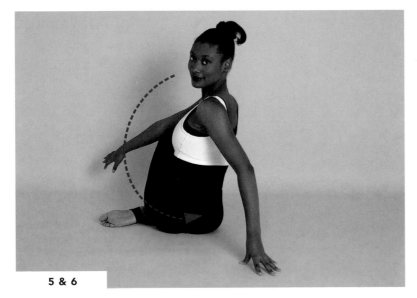

5 & 6

moving
routines

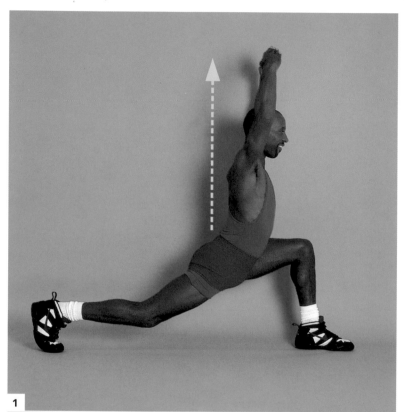

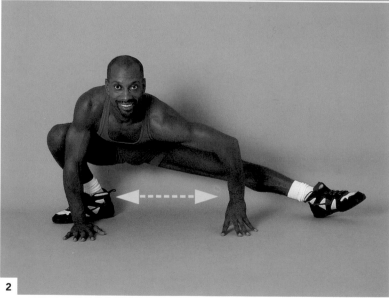

These routines combine basic stretches into flowing sequences that really give you a feeling for the way your body can move. Don't forget to use music to inspire you!

BOOKENDS

This is a short moving routine that takes you through many of the basic stretching moves for legs and groin. Ease into each stretch gently and try to make all your movements as calm as possible. The transitions from one move to the next should be especially easy and smooth. Use music to help your movements flow and to reflect your mood.

POSITION 1:

Start in an upright position, facing the side of your room, and give yourself a quick posture check (see page 25). Now lift both arms to the ceiling, stretching up high and elongating the spine. Keeping your arms raised, slowly start to reach one leg back behind you into a low lunge. Keep the weight over your front leg as you stretch the other leg behind – this will help you keep your balance – and only settle the weight equally on both feet once you have your back leg behind you.
• Stretches groin and hamstrings.

POSITION 2:

From your lunge position, bring your arms down to rest your hands on the floor for support, either side of

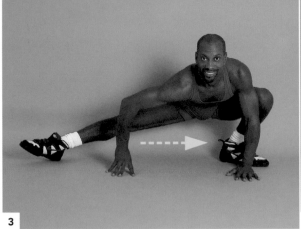

3

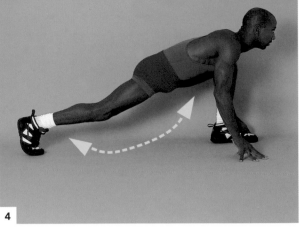

4

the bent leg. Then bring the arms in front of the bent leg and swivel to face the front of the room, keeping one leg bent and the other straight. This involves pressing the leg of the bent knee back as you turn in your hip. Your final position should be as in the photograph, with both arms in front of the legs and both heels ideally touching the ground.

• This mobilizes the hip area and stretches the inner thigh muscles.

POSITION 3:

Using your hands and the strength in your legs, simply push yourself over to the other side so that you end

with the other leg bent, in a mirror image of position 2. Keep your backside and hips low to the ground as you swing across to the other side. This movement should feel smooth and unrestricted and you will feel more stretch in those inner thighs as you move. Keeping the hands on the floor will support you, but as you get stronger and more flexible, try reaching your hands out in front of you so that all the work is done in the legs.

POSITION 4:

From your side lunge, turn back into a forward facing lunge (you will now

be facing the opposite direction to where you started), resting fingertips on the floor. Once again you are swivelling in the hip and coming to rest in a low lunge.

• Stretches out the groin area.

POSITION 5:

Keeping the left hip pressed forward, drop the knee of the back leg to the floor. Rest here a moment to feel an added stretch on the front of that thigh and then bend up the back leg. Reach your hand behind you to grasp the upturned foot and pull it towards your backside. Hold for 15 seconds.

• Puts a real stretch on the front of that back leg, which you should feel right up your torso.

Once you are at ease in this last position (and it is quite an advanced stretch), your sense of balance will improve. You could even try taking your front hand off the floor and posing! This is your bookend position, which calls for balance and flexibility at the same time.

• Don't forget to repeat the whole sequence going the other way, so that you end up stretching the other thigh.

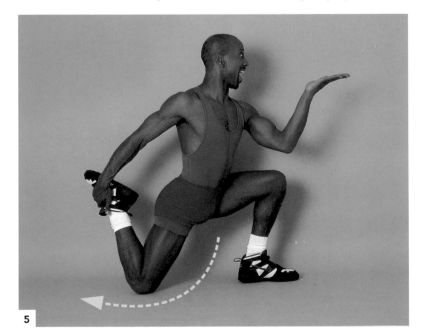

5

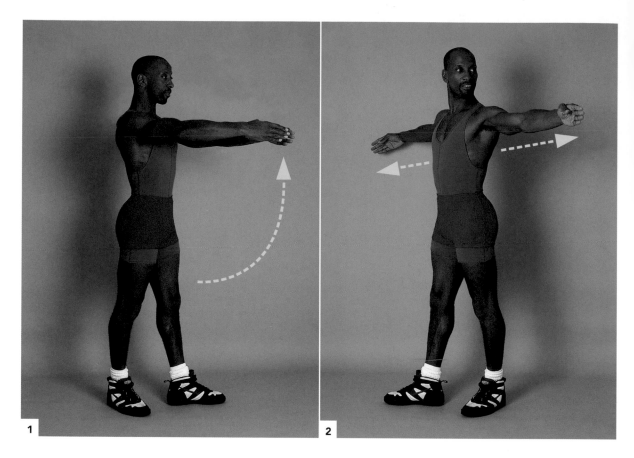

1   **2**

"GET EMOTIONAL!"

This is your chance to put some real feeling into your movement routine. It is a simple stretch routine that you can learn easily and then interpret so that it is matched to your own ability and mood.

Use the moves to express what you are feeling, whether it is frustration or joy. As you move your arms or legs, follow their path with your eyes and really extend your movements, sending the movement beyond your own body.

Put some stirring music on, find a place where you can be alone and really get into it – express yourself! You'll be surprised at how liberating and relaxing the experience is.

POSITION 1:

Start out standing tall, with the weight equally on both feet. After checking your posture (see page 25), slowly draw both arms up in front of you. As you raise the arms, try to imagine that the lift is coming right through the spine, making you so much taller that the top of your head presses against the ceiling.

Keep the arms "soft" – that is, not straight but slightly rounded, with fingertips just touching. The torso should be lifted via the abdominals but not held rigid but relaxed, with the shoulder blades pressed down. Relax the facial muscles and think about sending the energy out well beyond your fingertips.

POSITION 2:

Still keeping the arms relaxed and soft, follow your hands with your eyes as the arms part and open to a wide position that you can hold for a moment or two. Feel the muscles of the chest expanding as you press your arms open and put some strength into the motion, opening your arms and sending the energy out through the ends of each finger.

Now take both arms up above your head, palms back to back, still following the hands with your eyes so that the back starts to arch slightly as you look upwards. Keep the torso lifted as you arch so that there is no pressure on the lower back.

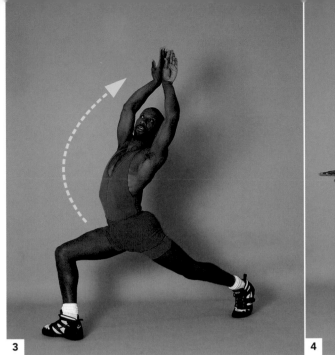

3

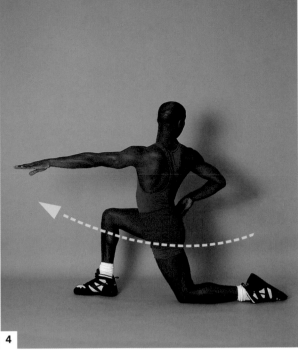

4

POSITION 3:

From this arched position with the arms lifted, slide one leg back and bend your front leg into a low lunge position. Feel the stretch under the groin area.

• This pose stretches the groin and the back of the legs.

POSITION 4:

Once into the lunge, drop your back knee to the floor and, keeping the hips pressed forwards, twist the upper body to look behind you. Open up the arms from above your head and use them to help you twist, pulling the back hand onto the hip.

Turn your head to follow the line of your twist and gaze ahead.

• Mobilizes the waist and stretches the groin and the front of the back thigh.

POSITION 5:

The grand finale – untwist the torso so that your bent arm comes back towards the front. Circle your right arm up in front, over your head and back behind you so that you can lean back and put your weight on it. To do this you must arch your back and push the hips forwards. With the other arm, make a half circle that reaches upwards to the sky in an emotive ending! The back is in as deep an arch as is comfortable, with one arm supporting you and the other stretching upwards.

Try this whole routine with the other leg, so that you feel the stretch on the other side. And don't forget that the more often you do this, the easier it will become and the more emotion you can put into it!

• Mobilizes the shoulders, back and hips.

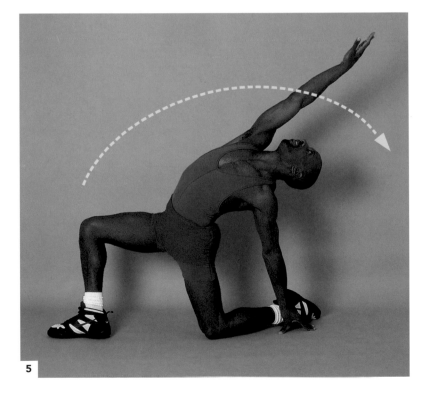

5

stretch index

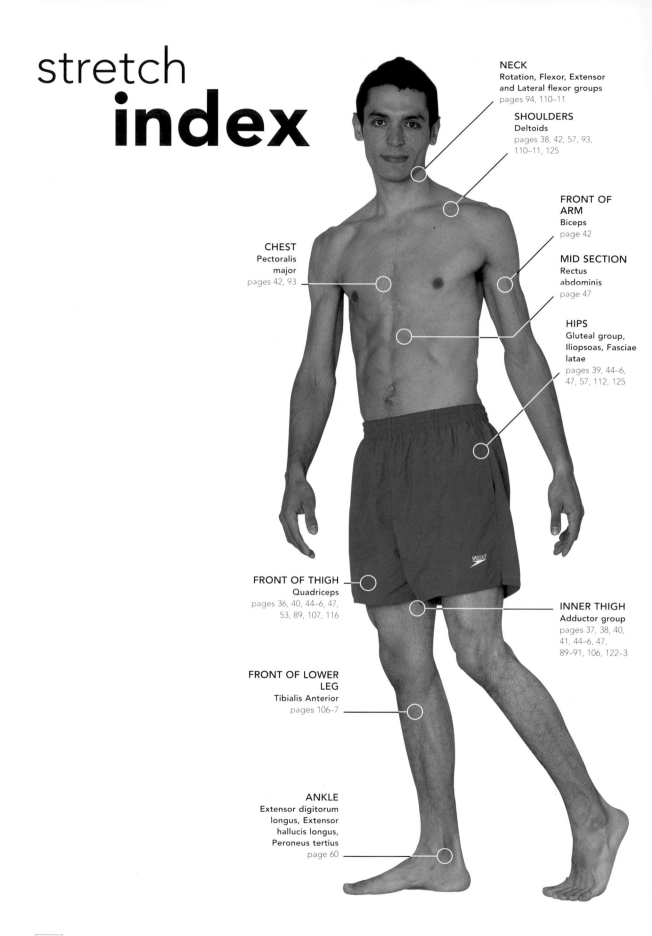

NECK
Rotation, Flexor, Extensor and Lateral flexor groups
pages 94, 110–11

SHOULDERS
Deltoids
pages 38, 42, 57, 93, 110–11, 125

FRONT OF ARM
Biceps
page 42

MID SECTION
Rectus abdominis
page 47

CHEST
Pectoralis major
pages 42, 93

HIPS
Gluteal group, Iliopsoas, Fasciae latae
pages 39, 44–6, 47, 57, 112, 125

FRONT OF THIGH
Quadriceps
pages 36, 40, 44–6, 47, 53, 89, 107, 116

INNER THIGH
Adductor group
pages 37, 38, 40, 41, 44–6, 47, 89–91, 106, 122–3

FRONT OF LOWER LEG
Tibialis Anterior
pages 106–7

ANKLE
Extensor digitorum longus, Extensor hallucis longus, Peroneus tertius
page 60

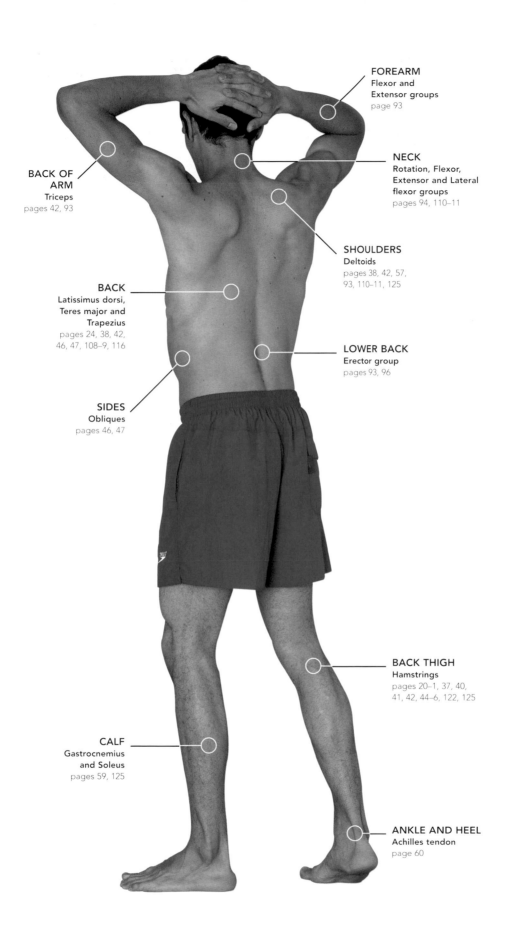

FOREARM
Flexor and
Extensor groups
page 93

NECK
Rotation, Flexor,
Extensor and Lateral
flexor groups
pages 94, 110–11

BACK OF
ARM
Triceps
pages 42, 93

SHOULDERS
Deltoids
pages 38, 42, 57,
93, 110–11, 125

BACK
Latissimus dorsi,
Teres major and
Trapezius
pages 24, 38, 42,
46, 47, 108–9, 116

LOWER BACK
Erector group
pages 93, 96

SIDES
Obliques
pages 46, 47

BACK THIGH
Hamstrings
pages 20–1, 37, 40,
41, 42, 44–6, 122, 125

CALF
Gastrocnemius
and Soleus
pages 59, 125

ANKLE AND HEEL
Achilles tendon
page 60

Index